VARIATION IN HEALTH CARE SPENDING

Target Decision Making, Not Geography

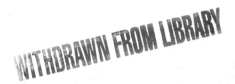
Committee on Geographic Variation in Health Care
Spending and Promotion of High-Value Care

Board on Health Care Services

Joseph P. Newhouse, Alan M. Garber, Robin P. Graham,
Margaret A. McCoy, Michelle Mancher, and Ashna Kibria, *Editors*

INSTITUTE OF MEDICINE
OF THE NATIONAL ACADEMIES

THE NATIONAL ACADEMIES PRESS
Washington, D.C.
www.nap.edu

1900978

MAR 1 4 2014

THE NATIONAL ACADEMIES PRESS   500 Fifth Street, NW   Washington, DC 20001

NOTICE: The project that is the subject of this report was approved by the Governing Board of the National Research Council, whose members are drawn from the councils of the National Academy of Sciences, the National Academy of Engineering, and the Institute of Medicine. The members of the committee responsible for the report were chosen for their special competences and with regard for appropriate balance.

This study was supported by Contract/Grant No. HHSP23320042509XI between the National Academy of Sciences and the Centers for Medicare & Medicaid Services, Department of Health and Human Services. Any opinions, findings, conclusions, or recommendations expressed in this publication are those of the editors and do not necessarily reflect the views of the organizations or agencies that provided support for the project.

International Standard Book Number-13: 978-0-309-28869-9
International Standard Book Number-10: 0-309-28869-X

Additional copies of this report are available for sale from the National Academies Press, 500 Fifth Street, NW, Keck 360, Washington, DC 20001; (800) 624-6242 or (202) 334-3313; http://www.nap.edu.

For more information about the Institute of Medicine, visit the IOM home page at: **www.iom.edu.**

The serpent has been a symbol of long life, healing, and knowledge among almost all cultures and religions since the beginning of recorded history. The serpent adopted as a logotype by the Institute of Medicine is a relief carving from ancient Greece, now held by the Staatliche Museen in Berlin.

Suggested citation: IOM (Institute of Medicine). 2013. *Variation in health care spending: Target decision making, not geography.* Washington, DC: The National Academies Press.

"Knowing is not enough; we must apply.
Willing is not enough; we must do."
—Goethe

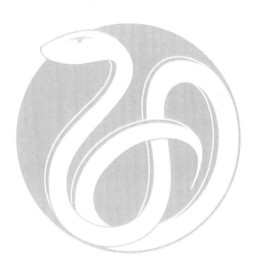

INSTITUTE OF MEDICINE
OF THE NATIONAL ACADEMIES

Advising the Nation. Improving Health.

THE NATIONAL ACADEMIES
Advisers to the Nation on Science, Engineering, and Medicine

The **National Academy of Sciences** is a private, nonprofit, self-perpetuating society of distinguished scholars engaged in scientific and engineering research, dedicated to the furtherance of science and technology and to their use for the general welfare. Upon the authority of the charter granted to it by the Congress in 1863, the Academy has a mandate that requires it to advise the federal government on scientific and technical matters. Dr. Ralph J. Cicerone is president of the National Academy of Sciences.

The **National Academy of Engineering** was established in 1964, under the charter of the National Academy of Sciences, as a parallel organization of outstanding engineers. It is autonomous in its administration and in the selection of its members, sharing with the National Academy of Sciences the responsibility for advising the federal government. The National Academy of Engineering also sponsors engineering programs aimed at meeting national needs, encourages education and research, and recognizes the superior achievements of engineers. Dr. C. D. Mote, Jr., is president of the National Academy of Engineering.

The **Institute of Medicine** was established in 1970 by the National Academy of Sciences to secure the services of eminent members of appropriate professions in the examination of policy matters pertaining to the health of the public. The Institute acts under the responsibility given to the National Academy of Sciences by its congressional charter to be an adviser to the federal government and, upon its own initiative, to identify issues of medical care, research, and education. Dr. Harvey V. Fineberg is president of the Institute of Medicine.

The **National Research Council** was organized by the National Academy of Sciences in 1916 to associate the broad community of science and technology with the Academy's purposes of furthering knowledge and advising the federal government. Functioning in accordance with general policies determined by the Academy, the Council has become the principal operating agency of both the National Academy of Sciences and the National Academy of Engineering in providing services to the government, the public, and the scientific and engineering communities. The Council is administered jointly by both Academies and the Institute of Medicine. Dr. Ralph J. Cicerone and Dr. C. D. Mote, Jr., are chair and vice chair, respectively, of the National Research Council.

www.national-academies.org

THOMAS H. LEE, Professor of Medicine, Harvard Medical School and Harvard School of Public Health; CEO, Partners Community HealthCare, Inc., Boston, Massachusetts

MARK B. McCLELLAN, Director, Engelberg Center for Health Care Reform; Leonard D. Schaeffer Chair in Health Policy Studies, Brookings Institution, Washington, DC

SALLY C. MORTON, Professor and Chair, Department of Biostatistics, Graduate School of Public Health, University of Pittsburgh, Pennsylvania

ROBERT D. REISCHAUER, Distinguished Institute Fellow and President Emeritus, The Urban Institute, Washington, DC

ALAN WEIL, Executive Director, National Academy for State Health Policy, Washington, DC

GAIL R. WILENSKY, Senior Fellow, Project HOPE, Bethesda, Maryland

Study Staff

ROBIN P. GRAHAM, Senior Program Officer, Study Director
DIANNE WOLMAN, Senior Program Officer (through December 2010)
MARGARET A. McCOY, Program Officer
MEG F. BARRY, Associate Program Officer (through December 2012)
MICHELLE MANCHER, Associate Program Officer
ASHNA KIBRIA, Research Associate (from July 2012)
CASSANDRA CACACE, Research Associate (October 2011 through April 2012)
REBECCA MARKSAMER, Research Associate (from February 2013)
NINA SURESH, Research Assistant (through August 2012)
JILLIAN LAFFREY, Assistant, Board on Health Care Services
KATERINA HORSKA, Presidential Management Fellow (December 2011 through May 2012)
MARGARET L. SCHWARZE, IOM Anniversary Fellow
SETH GLICKMAN, IOM Anniversary Fellow
ROGER HERDMAN, Director, Board on Health Care Services

Consultants

GARY ALLEN, Truven Health Analytics
ABBY ALPERT, RAND Corporation
DAVID AUERBACH, RAND Corporation
ANITA AU-YEUNG, Acumen, LLC
SARAH AXEEN, Precision Health Economics
KATHERINE BAICKER, Harvard University
SEO HYON BAIK, University of Pittsburgh

JOHN BAILAR, University of Chicago (Emeritus)
ERIC BARRETTE, The Lewin Group
HANI BASHOUR, Acumen, LLC
JAY BHATTACHARYA, Acumen, LLC
RONA BRIERE, Technical Writing Consultant
AMITABH CHANDRA, Harvard Kennedy School of Government
MICHAEL CHERNEW, Department of Health Care Policy, Harvard
    Medical School
CAMILLE CHICKLIS, Acumen, LLC
KENNAN CRONEN, Acumen, LLC
BRYAN DOWD, University of Minnesota
EMILY EHRLICH, Truven Health Analytics
AMANDA FARR, Truven Health Analytics
ELLIOTT S. FISHER, Dartmouth Institute for Health Policy and Clinical
    Practice
CAROL FORHAN, Truven Health Analytics
JESSELYN FRILEY, Acumen, LLC
PROJESH GHOSH, The Lewin Group
TERESA GIBSON, Department of Health Care Policy, Harvard Medical
    School; Truven Health Analytics
IAN GLENN, The Lewin Group
DANA GOLDMAN, Precision Health Economics
CLIFFORD GOODMAN, The Lewin Group
DANIEL GOTTLIEB, Dartmouth Institute for Health Policy and Clinical
    Practice
THOMAS HOERGER, RTI International
PAUL HOGAN, The Lewin Group
PETER HUCKFELDT, RAND Corporation
MARCO D. HUESCH, University of Southern California
PETER HUSSEY, RAND Corporation
JOSIE IDOKO, The Lewin Group
MELINA IMSHAUG, Truven Health Analytics
CAMERON KAPLAN, University of Pittsburgh
DARIUS LAKDAWALLA, Precision Health Economics
BRUCE LANDON, Department of Health Care Policy, Harvard Medical
    School; Division of Primary Care and General Internal Medicine,
    Department of Medicine, Beth Israel Deaconess Medical Center
MARY BETH LANDRUM, Department of Health Care Policy, Harvard
    Medical School
CHRISTOPHER LAU, RAND Corporation
BRANDY LIPTON, Acumen, LLC
HANGSHENG LIU, RAND Corporation
THOMAS MaCURDY, Acumen, LLC

WILLARD G. MANNING, University of Chicago
JACLYN MARSHALL, The Lewin Group
MICHAEL McKELLAR, Department of Health Care Policy, Harvard Medical School
ELLEN MEARA, Dartmouth Institute for Health Policy and Clinical Practice
ATEEV MEHROTRA, RAND Corporation
COURT MELIN, The Lewin Group
KAY MILLER, Truven Health Analytics
BRIAN MOORE, Truven Health Analytics
CAITLIN MORRIS, The Lewin Group
SIVIA NAIMER, Department of Health Care Policy, Harvard Medical School
SEBASTIAN NEGRUSA, The Lewin Group
SIMON NEUWAHL, RTI International
EDWARD C. NORTON, University of Michigan
MICHAEL K. ONG, University of California, Los Angeles
DANIELLA PERLROTH, Acumen, LLC
TOMAS PHILIPSON, Precision Health Economics
BRADY POST, The Lewin Group
DANIEL ROGERS, Acumen, LLC
JOHN ROMLEY, Precision Health Economics
SHAHIN SANEINEJAD, Acumen, LLC
JASON SHAFRIN, Acumen, LLC
VICTORIA SHIER, RAND Corporation
ELEN SHRESTHA, Acumen, LLC
JONATHAN SKINNER, Dartmouth Institute for Health Policy and Clinical Practice
MARK TOTTEN, RAND Corporation
JASON WAHLMAN, The Lewin Group
NANCY WALCZAK, The Lewin Group
JOHN WARNER, The Lewin Group
ADAM S. WILK, University of Michigan
BENJAMIN YARNOFF, RTI International
SAJID ZAIDI, Acumen, LLC
YUTING ZHANG, University of Pittsburgh
WEIPING ZHOU, Dartmouth Institute for Health Policy and Clinical Practice

Reviewers

This report has been reviewed in draft form by individuals chosen for their diverse perspectives and technical expertise, in accordance with procedures approved by the National Research Council's Report Review Committee. The purpose of this independent review is to provide candid and critical comments that will assist the institution in making its published report as sound as possible and to ensure that the report meets institutional standards for objectivity, evidence, and responsiveness to the study charge. The review comments and draft manuscript remain confidential to protect the integrity of the deliberative process. We wish to thank the following individuals for their review of this report:

HENRY AARON, The Brookings Institution
STUART ALTMAN, Brandeis University
GERARD F. ANDERSON, Johns Hopkins University
DAVID A. ASCH, University of Pennsylvania
KATHERINE BAICKER, Harvard School of Public Health
RICHARD A. BERMAN, Emeritus, Manhattanville College
DAVID BLUMENTHAL, The Commonwealth Fund
ELLIOT FISHER, Dartmouth Institute of Health Policy and Clinical Practice
ELIZABETH A. McGLYNN, Kaiser Permanente
MARILYN MOON, American Institutes for Research
ROBERT PHILLIPS, American Academy of Family Physicians
THOMAS M. PRISELAC, Cedars-Sinai Health System
JOHN ROTHER, National Coalition on Health Care

DANA GELB SAFRAN, Blue Cross Blue Shield of Massachusetts
GORDON TRAPNELL, Actuarial Research Corporation
ALAN M. ZASLAVSKY, Harvard Medical School
STEVE ZUCKERMAN, The Urban Institute

Although the reviewers listed above provided many constructive comments and suggestions, they were not asked to endorse the report's observations nor did they see the final draft of the report before its release. The review of this report was overseen by **DONALD M. STEINWACHS,** Johns Hopkins Institute for Policy Studies, and **CHARLES E. PHELPS,** University of Rochester (Emeritus). Appointed by the Institute of Medicine and the National Research Council, they were responsible for making certain that an independent examination of this report was carried out in accordance with institutional procedures and that all review comments were carefully considered. Responsibility for the final content of this report rests entirely with the authoring committee and the institution.

Foreword

Medicare's current cost trajectory is unsustainable. However, cutting expenditures through indiscriminate payment or benefit reductions would tend to shift costs to overburdened beneficiaries or diminish access to and quality of care. The only sensible way to restrain costs is to enhance the value of the health care system, thus extracting more benefit from the dollars spent. Public officials and policy makers long have searched for a simple way to accomplish this task and recently proposed an approach based on the long-standing phenomenon of geographic variation in Medicare spending and quality. The underlying premise is that certain regions of the United States spend less per Medicare beneficiary because they are more efficient providers of health care. If only researchers were able to determine what these high-value regions do that low-value ones do not, the theory goes, the core goal of the U.S. health care system (simultaneous achievement of high performance and affordability) could be achieved.

The Institute of Medicine's Committee on Geographic Variation in Health Care Spending and Promotion of High-Value Care explored a wealth of public (Medicare and Medicaid) and private (commercial insurer) data to understand better the extent and sources of geographic variation in spending and quality for Medicare and for the U.S. health care system as a whole. The data informing the committee's work may be accessed at www.iom.edu/geovariationmaterials. The analyses of these data exposed a number of new questions, as well as answers. Do existing measures of health status account sufficiently for differences in disease burden among regions? How does one adequately measure market competition, let alone patient preferences and provider discretion? Do the geographic regions

xi

studied represent the health care markets where most health care spending occurs for respective regional populations?

In its critical and comprehensive assessment, the committee uncovered layers of complexity: Variation exists not only across previously defined geographies, but also among hospital service areas within them, across health service sectors and clinical condition categories, and for individual providers. There is no clear pattern suggesting that certain regions or providers uniformly deliver higher-value care than others. This conclusion implies that sound solutions for achieving high-value care should be derived from, and targeted to, the loci of health care decisions, including hospitals, single- and multispecialty physician groups, health care organizations, and individual practitioners and patients. The Center for Medicare and Medicaid Innovation is mandated by the Patient Protection and Affordable Care Act to support innovative payment and organizational models that target a variety of health care decision makers. Fulfilling this mandate is one way the United States can test and evaluate different payment reform models to identify those that influence decisions about care delivery most constructively.

I would like to thank the committee and staff who undertook this formidable assessment and produced a straightforward and concise report that illuminates the relationship between variation in health care spending and the promotion of high-value care.

Harvey V. Fineberg
President, Institute of Medicine

Preface

Variation in medical practice has undoubtedly existed for centuries. The modern era of interest in geographic variation in health care began with a 1938 publication by Sir Alison Glover, which reported that tonsillectomies were performed at widely varying rates across different locations in England. This report, and others that followed, revealed not only that physicians varied in how they treated apparently similar patients, but also that their patterns of treatment clustered geographically. This variation is now known to be a feature of almost every country's health care system. In the United States, the efforts of a dedicated group of researchers at Dartmouth Medical School have raised awareness of the phenomenon of geographic variation in health care among professionals, government officials and legislators, and the public. The Dartmouth researchers began by defining market areas within the United States and examining variation in practice across those areas using data from the original Medicare program. For many years they have published the *Dartmouth Atlas of Health Care*, documenting in great and colorful detail the large variation in both spending and service utilization exhibited by these market areas.

This variation attracted additional attention from members of Congress after Medicare Part C, now known as Medicare Advantage, was established in the 1980s. Because payment to the health plans that participated in Part C was based on spending for traditional Medicare in the beneficiary's county of residence, and because that spending varied, payments to Part C health plans varied widely across areas. This variation in turn led to more generous supplementary benefits, lower cost sharing, and lower premiums in the high-spending areas. Members of Congress from the lower-spending areas began to question why their constituents did not receive the same benefits as residents of the high-spending areas, and they asked how per-beneficiary expenditures could vary so greatly in a federal program that was ostensibly uniform throughout the nation.

These observations and questions led to proposals for creating a value index to reallocate Medicare spending. A value index would adjust Medicare reimbursement in an area according to the area's value of services, rewarding areas that provided high-quality services at relatively low cost. The committee that produced this report was asked to address the desirability of such an index, and it did so in an interim report issued in March 2013.

Because the committee was charged with an ambitious set of goals that went well beyond consideration of a value index, it conducted a broad inquiry into geographic variation. First, it looked at spending in Medicare Parts C and D by area, not just the spending in the traditional Medicare program that has been exhibited in the *Dartmouth Atlas*. The proportion of Medicare beneficiaries in an area enrolled in Part C varies widely across the country; to the degree that beneficiaries in Part C have different health risks from those in the original Medicare program, including them could yield a different picture of total Medicare spending. The same is true of Medicare Part D. Although dollar spending under Part D is considerably smaller than that under Parts A and B, it does not exhibit the same geographic patterns.

Second, because Medicare accounts for only a minority of health care spending in an area, the committee tried to estimate the total spending in an area by all payers. Hospitals, physicians, and other health care providers treat both Medicare and non-Medicare patients, so their economic conditions and the incentives they face are influenced by commercial insurers and other payers, not Medicare alone. A hospital's nursing staff, for example, treats all the hospital's patients, not just its Medicare patients, and in considering the quantity and quality of nursing staff to hire, the hospital will take account of its revenue from all payers. This is obviously the case for its capital spending as well. Moreover, Medicare beneficiaries use a different mix of services from those used by the nonelderly population, which could result in a different spending pattern.

Estimates of total spending are necessarily limited by the data available. Although the Medical Expenditure Panel Survey obtains data on spending by all payers, it is not large enough to provide reliable estimates of such spending for each market, nor is that its intent. There is no data source for commercial claims or Medicaid comparable to the large database of Medicare health care claims that can be used to quantify spending at the market level. The committee was able, however, to contract for analyses of two very large commercial databases. Although neither of these databases is a random sample of all Americans with commercial insurance, the results of these two analyses are largely, though not entirely, consistent, giving the committee confidence that it could draw reasonable inferences about commercial spending in each area. The committee's estimates for Medicaid and the uninsured are even less precise than those for the commercially insured, but the committee believes it has done the best job possible with existing data to quantify the variation in total spending across geographic areas.

Unusual for an Institute of Medicine committee, this committee had a substantial research budget with which to conduct original empirical analyses. But the ability to direct the data collection and analyses that this budget enabled was only one reason that it was a pleasure for us to chair this endeavor. The committee itself was outstanding and worked together harmoniously to assess, analyze, and draw conclusions from the vast array of numbers that the subcontractors commissioned to conduct these analyses produced at the committee's request. We also wish to thank the staff who worked long hours to coordinate the activities of the many subcontractors and to translate the committee's deliberations into prose, as well as the subcontractors, whose results deeply informed the thinking that is documented in this report.

Joseph P. Newhouse, *Chair*
Alan M. Garber, *Vice-Chair*
Committee on Geographic Variation in Health
Care Spending and Promotion of High-Value Care

Acknowledgments

The committee and staff are indebted to a number of individuals and organizations for their contributions to this report. The following individuals provided testimony to the committee at its public sessions:

Jeffrey Bailet, Aurora Medical Group

Donald M. Berwick, Former President and CEO, Institute for Healthcare Improvement

Jonathan Blum, Centers for Medicare & Medicaid Services

Carolyn Clancy, Director, Agency for Healthcare Research and Quality

Janet Corrigan, National Quality Forum

Denis Cortese, Arizona State University

Helen Darling, National Business Group on Health

William Davenhall, Department of Health and Human Services, Esri

Chris Dawe, Committee on Finance, U.S. Senate

Larry DeGhetaldi, California Medical Association

Cynthia Flynn, Family Health and Birth Center

Geoff Gerhardt, Subcommittee on Health, Committee on Ways and Means, U.S. House of Representatives

Raymond Gibbons, Mayo Clinic

Elizabeth Gilbertson, Hotel Employees and Restaurant Employees International Union Welfare Fund

Timothy Gronniger, Committee on Energy and Commerce, U.S. House of Representatives

Lorrie Kaplan, American College of Nurse-Midwives

Michael Kitchell, Iowa Medical Society
Richard Kronick, Office of the Assistant Secretary for Planning and
    Evaluation
Nancy Lane, PDA Inc. Health Planning Management Consultants
John (Jack) Lewin, American College of Cardiology
Scott Malaney, American Hospital Association
Mark Miller, Medicare Payment Advisory Commission
Larry Minnix, American Association of Homes and Services for the
    Aging
Sam Nussbaum, WellPoint
Peggy O'Kane, National Committee for Quality Assurance
Anne O'Rourke, California Hospital Association
Herbert Pardes, New York Presbyterian Hospital
Bruce Pyenson, Milliman, Inc.
Chris Queram, Wisconsin Collaborative for Healthcare Quality
William Rich, American Academy of Ophthalmology
Michael Richards, Gundersen Lutheran Health System
James Rohack, Scott & White Center for Healthcare Policy
Craig Samitt, Dean Clinic
Deborah Schumann, Physicians for a National Health Program
The Honorable Allyson Schwartz, U.S. House of Representatives
    (D-PA)
Jason Scull, Infectious Disease Society of America
Eileen Sullivan-Marx, University of Pennsylvania School of Nursing
Jonathan Sunshine, American College of Radiology
John Tooker, American College of Physicians
Karl Ulrich, Marshfield Clinic
Susan Walden, Health Policy Counsel, Committee on Finance
    (Minority), U.S. Senate
Lina Walker, AARP
Andrea Weddle, HIV Medicine Association

We also extend special thanks to the following individuals who were essential sources of information, generously giving their time and knowledge
to further the committee's efforts:

Arlene S. Ash, University of Massachusetts Medical School
Alan D. Aviles, New York City Health and Hospitals Corporation
John Bertko, Centers for Medicare & Medicaid Services
Mark S. Blumberg, MD, TruRisk LLC
Congressman Earl Blumenauer, State of Oregon
Rick Cooper, CEO, The Everett Clinic
Guy David, University of Pennsylvania

Mark Duggan, Wharton School, University of Pennsylvania
Abe Dunn, Bureau of Economic Analysis
Anne Elixhauser, Agency for Healthcare Research and Quality
Sherry Glied, Columbia University, Mailman School of Public Health
Senator Chuck Grassley, State of Iowa
Atul Grover, Association of American Medical Colleges
James H. Harrison, Onpoint Health Data
Christine L. Johnson, Florida Hospital Association
Abbi Kaplan, Washington Healthcare Forum
Lorrie Kline Kaplan, American College of Nurse-Midwives
Bruce M. Kelly, Mayo Clinic
Robert Krasowski, National Center for Health Statistics/Research
    Data Center
Congressman Rick Larsen, State of Washington
Roderick J. Little, University of Michigan
Willard G. Manning, Emeritus, The University of Chicago
Peter McMenamin, American Nurses Association
Nancy McNeilly, National Association of Urban Hospitals
Karen Milgate, Centers for Medicare & Medicaid Services
Mark Miller, Medicare Payment Advisory Commission
Arielle Mir, Medicare Payment Advisory Commission
Robert Murray, Maryland Department of Health and Mental
    Hygiene
Edward C. Norton, University of Michigan School of Public Health
Wendell Primus, Senior Policy Advisor, Office of the House Minority
    Leader
Chris Mambu Rasch, Wisconsin Medical Society
Dana Gelb Safran, Blue Cross Blue Shield of Massachusetts
Deborah Schumann, Physicians for a National Health Program
James G. Scott, Applied Policy
Frank A. Sloan, Duke University
Caroline Steinberg, American Hospital Association
Jeffrey Stensland, Medicare Payment Advisory Commission
Mayor Ray Stephanson, Everett, Washington
David Wennberg, The Dartmouth Institute
John E. Wennberg, The Dartmouth Institute

We would like to thank OptumInsight for the use of the Normative Health Information database, the Centers for Medicare & Medicaid Services (CMS) and Truven Health Analytics for providing new data on geographic variation, and Verisk Health for making the DxCG® DCG Commercial Software available to our contractors. Their contributions to our research were substantial and essential. We would also like to thank Rona Briere for her expert assistance in editing the report and Alisa Decatur for her support in manuscript preparation.

Funding for this study was provided by the CMS. The committee appreciates the opportunity and support extended by CMS for the development of this report.

Finally, many individuals within the Institute of Medicine were helpful to the study staff. We would like to thank Clyde Behney, Laura Harbold DeStefano, Chelsea Frakes, Jim Jensen, Sandra McDermin, William McLeod, Abbey Meltzer, Christine Stencel, Vilija Teel, Lauren Tobias, Cheryl Ulmer, Jennifer Walsh, and Sarah Ziegenhorn.

Contents

Abstract

For more than three decades, experts at the Dartmouth Institute for Health Policy and Clinical Practice have documented that Medicare spending varies greatly across geographic regions, and that higher expenditures do not correspond to better health care outcomes. This seminal body of work raised the possibility that some regions of the country may be more efficient than others at providing high-quality health care services. Seeking strategies for reducing Medicare costs, some wonder whether cutting payment rates to high-cost areas would save money without adversely affecting health care quality for Medicare beneficiaries. This Institute of Medicine study was undertaken to independently evaluate geographic variation in health care spending levels and growth among Medicare, Medicaid, privately insured, and uninsured populations in the United States; to make recommendations for changes in Medicare payment systems under the Patient Protection and Affordable Care Act (ACA); and to address whether Medicare payments for physicians and hospitals should be adjusted by a value index that is based on geographic area performance.

This report presents findings from commissioned analyses of traditional, fee-for-service Medicare (and to a lesser extent Medicare Advantage, or Part C) and commercial insurance. Because of methodological challenges and data limitations, it does not include separate analyses of variation in the Medicaid and uninsured populations, although estimates of spending by these two groups are included in the study committee's area-wide estimates of total health care spending. The commissioned analyses and the committee's research and deliberations led to the following conclusions:

- Geographic variation in spending and utilization is real, and not an artifact reflecting random noise; it persists across geographic units and health care services and over time.
- Variation in spending in the commercial insurance market is due mainly to differences in price markups by providers rather than to differences in the utilization of health care services.
- After accounting for differences in the age, sex, and health status of beneficiaries, geographic variation in spending in both Medicare and commercial insurance is not further explained by other beneficiary demographic factors, insurance plan factors, or market-level characteristics. In fact, after controlling for all factors measurable within the data used for this analysis, a large amount of variation remains unexplained.
- Total spending per Medicare beneficiary and per person with commercial insurance is little correlated across hospital referral regions (HRRs); utilization of services between the two populations, however, is much more correlated across HRRs.
- Health care decision making generally occurs at the level of the individual practitioner or organization (e.g., hospital or physician group), not at the level of a geographic region. Therefore, a geographically based value index is unlikely to promote more efficient behaviors among individual providers and thus is unlikely to improve the overall value of health care.
- Substantial variation in spending and utilization remains as units of analysis get progressively smaller (hospital referral region, hospital service area, hospital, practice, and individual provider).
- HRR-level quality is not consistently related to spending or utilization among either Medicare beneficiaries or the commercially insured.

The committee's first recommendation reflects research and data limitations encountered during the course of this study:

RECOMMENDATION 1: Congress should encourage the Centers for Medicare & Medicaid Services (CMS), and provide the necessary resources, to make accessing Medicare and Medicaid data easier for research purposes. CMS should collaborate with private insurers to collect, integrate, and analyze standardized data on spending, as well as clinical and behavioral health outcomes, to enable more extensive comparisons of payments and quality and evaluation of value-based payment models across payers.

The committee's remaining recommendations are based on the conclusions presented above and the committee's analysis of payment and organizational reforms that would promote the delivery of high-value care while taking account of the ACA and related changes already under way:

RECOMMENDATION 2: Congress should not adopt a geographically based value index for Medicare. Because geographic units are not where most health care decisions are made, a geographic value index would be a poorly targeted mechanism for encouraging value improvement. Adjusting payments geographically, based on any aggregate or composite measure of spending or quality, would unfairly reward low-value providers in high-value regions and punish high-value providers in low-value regions.

RECOMMENDATION 3: To improve value, the Centers for Medicare & Medicaid Services (CMS) should continue to test payment reforms that incentivize the clinical and financial integration of health care delivery systems and thereby encourage their (1) coordination of care among individual providers, (2) real-time sharing of data and tracking of service use and health outcomes, (3) receipt and distribution of provider payments, and (4) assumption of some or all of the risk of managing the care continuum for their populations. Further, CMS should pilot programs that allow beneficiaries to share in the savings due to higher-value care.

RECOMMENDATION 4: During the transition to new payment models, the Centers for Medicare & Medicaid Services (CMS) should conduct ongoing evaluations of the impact on value of the reforms included in Recommendation 3 by measuring Medicare spending and beneficiaries' clinical health outcomes. CMS should use the results of these evaluations to iteratively improve these payment models. CMS should also monitor how these reforms impact Medicare beneficiaries' access to medical care.

RECOMMENDATION 5: If evaluations of specific payment reforms demonstrate increased value, Congress should give the Centers for Medicare & Medicaid Services the flexibility to accelerate the transition from traditional Medicare to new payment models.

Summary

For more than three decades, experts at the Dartmouth Institute for Health Policy and Clinical Practice have documented significant variation in Medicare spending across geographic regions apparently unrelated to health care outcomes achieved. From this seminal body of work, an idea emerged that certain regions of the country may be uniformly more efficient than others at providing high-quality health care services. Moreover, many argue that Medicare's traditional fee-for-service reimbursement system is a major driver of both variation and waste in health care because it rewards providers based on the volume and intensity rather than the value of services delivered. Seeking strategies for reducing Medicare costs, some wonder whether cutting payment rates to high-cost areas would save money without adversely affecting health care quality for Medicare beneficiaries.

Other health care policy experts counter that supporters of the above policy proposal conflate the issue of improving value with that of reducing geographic variation. Some variation in health care spending is to be expected in an efficient health care system, reflecting "acceptable"—meaning driven by genuine health needs—differences in consumption of health care services by individual patients. Reducing geographic variation is desirable only to the extent that measured variation represents inefficiencies in the health care system. Further, the literature on geographic variation traditionally has focused on spending and utilization in fee-for-service Medicare. Little attention has been paid to Medicaid, the commercial health care sector, Medicare Advantage (also known as Part C), or the uninsured. Spending and utilization patterns in traditional Medicare should not be assumed to be representative of other populations or of total health care spending and utilization in the United States.

Still other health care policy experts argue that regionally based payments are inherently unfair and would fail to create market incentives necessary to promote high-value, patient-centered care. Furthermore, there may not exist a natural geographic unit to use in analyses of area variation, since inter-area variation remains substantial even when the areas are defined as smaller and smaller geographic units. In other words, intra-area variation can be large, and even larger than variation across areas. Finally, provider payments based on regional area performance would reward inefficient providers in low-cost regions and punish more efficient providers in high-cost regions.

STUDY CHARGE

In 2009, following negotiations related to passage of the Patient Protection and Affordable Care Act (ACA), a group of members of the U.S. House of Representatives known as the Quality Care Coalition asked Secretary of the Department of Health and Human Services (HHS) Kathleen Sebelius to sponsor two Institute of Medicine (IOM) studies focused on geographic payments under Medicare, independent of final health care reform legislation. The first study evaluated the accuracy of Medicare's geographic adjustment factors, which alter physician and hospital payment rates based on specific, geographically based input prices. The IOM released two related reports—*Geographic Adjustment in Medicare Payment—Phase 1: Improving Accuracy* and *Geographic Adjustment in Medicare Payment—Phase II: Implications for Access, Quality, and Efficiency*—in 2011 and 2012, respectively.

For the second study, documented in the present report, the Centers for Medicare & Medicaid Services (CMS) contracted with the IOM to conduct a 3-year consensus study under the guidance of a 19-member committee, focused on better understanding the relevance of geographic variation to payment policies designed to promote value across the U.S. health care system. The committee members included experts in health economics, statistics, health care financing, value-based health care purchasing, health services research, health law, and health disparities. The committee's statement of task draws on language in earlier federal health care reform legislation[1,2] and includes the following three tasks:

---

[1]Preservation of Access to Care for Medicare Beneficiaries and Pension Relief Act of 2010, Public Law 111-192, 111th Cong., 2nd sess. (June 25, 2010).

[2]The Affordable Health Care for America Act, H.R. 3962, 111th Cong., 1st sess. (October 29, 2009).

1. to independently evaluate geographic variation in health care spending levels and growth among Medicare, Medicaid, privately insured, and uninsured populations in the United States;
2. to make recommendations for changes in Medicare Part A, B, and C payments, considering findings from task 1, as well as changes to Medicare payment systems under the ACA; and
3. to address whether Medicare payments for physicians and hospitals should incorporate a value index that would modify the payments based on geographic area performance.

RESEARCH FRAMEWORK

To respond to its statement of task, the committee identified two basic questions:

1. What is known about geographic variation in health care spending, utilization, and quality?
2. Should geographically based measures of value be used to adjust Medicare fee-for-service hospital and provider reimbursement rates in a geographic region?

To help answer these questions and complement its review of the existing literature, the committee commissioned an extensive body of original empirical analyses of public and commercial databases and four papers from subject-matter experts, and held two public workshops. The empirical analyses were focused on describing and accounting for geographic variation in health care spending, utilization, and quality for the overall population, as well as for populations with specific diseases or conditions. The following seven subcontractors supported the committee's analytic work: Acumen, LLC; Dartmouth Institute of Health Policy and Clinical Practice; Harvard University; The Lewin Group; Precision Health Economics, LLC (PHE); RAND; and the University of Pittsburgh.

In accordance with its statement of task, the committee examined variation within "areas of different sizes" to determine how different levels of geographic aggregation affect variation. Consistent with prior literature, this study evaluates variation at the level of three area units of measurement: hospital service areas (HSAs), hospital referral regions (HRRs), and metropolitan core-based statistical areas (CBSAs, also known as metropolitan statistical areas [MSAs]). Box S-1 defines these units.

BOX S-1
Definitions of Geographic Units
Frequently Used in Health Services Research

- *Hospital service areas (HSAs)*—Created by Dartmouth and defined by assigning to an HSA the zip codes from which a hospital or several hospitals draw the greatest proportion of their Medicare patients. There are 3,426 HSAs.
- *Hospital referral regions (HRRs)*—Created by Dartmouth to represent regional health care markets for tertiary (complex) medical care. Dartmouth defined 306 HRRs by assigning HSAs to regions where the greatest proportion of major cardiovascular procedures were performed, "with minor modifications to achieve geographic contiguity, a minimum total population size of 120,000, and a high localization index."
- *Metropolitan statistical areas (MSAs, or metropolitan core-based statistical areas [CBSAs])*—Created by the Office of Management and Budget using counties. Each of 388 MSAs includes one or more counties with one core urban area of 50,000 individuals or more, as well as "adjacent counties exhibiting a high degree of social and economic integration" (as measured by such factors as commuting patterns) with an urban core. Areas that do not qualify as MSAs are often classified as "outside" MSAs or non-MSAs. The Centers for Medicare & Medicaid Services (CMS) adjusts hospital payments according to a hospital wage index calculated for MSAs and non-MSAs.*

---

*CBSAs are geographic entities that the Office of Management and Budget implemented in 2003. The committee's commissioned analyses used MSAs (a subcomponent of CBSAs also referred to as metropolitan CBSAs), as well as non-MSA "rest of state" regions. For simplicity, and in accordance with expert practice in this area, the committee uses the term "metropolitan CBSA" throughout this report.

EMPIRICAL ANALYSIS OF GEOGRAPHIC VARIATION

The subcontractors conducted a series of regression and correlation analyses to quantify geographic variation in spending, utilization, and quality across various populations, payers, and geographic units; evaluate known (and measurable) factors that account for variation; and identify the types of health care services with disproportionately high rates of variation that drive total variation. Specifically, the analyses examined the roles of such factors as patient health status and demographic characteristics, health plan, and price and market factors in accounting for geographic variation.

This report presents the committee's findings based primarily on the commissioned analyses of traditional, fee-for-service Medicare (and to a lesser extent Medicare Advantage, or Part C) and commercial insurance. It does not include separate analyses of variation in the Medicaid and uninsured populations, although estimates of spending by these two groups are included in the committee's area-wide estimates of total health care spending (see the related discussion in Chapter 2).

CONCLUSIONS

Conclusion 2.1.[3] *Geographic variation in spending and utilization is real, and not an artifact reflecting random noise. The committee's empirical analyses of Medicare and commercial data confirm the robust presence of variation, which persists across geographic units and health care services and over time.*

Prior research by Dartmouth researchers and by the Medicare Payment Advisory Commission (MedPAC) found that unadjusted Medicare spending per beneficiary is 50-55 percent higher in regions in the highest quintile of spending relative to those in the lowest quintile, while Medicare service utilization is approximately 30 percent greater in the highest quintile than in the lowest. These findings are corroborated by the committee's commissioned analyses, which show that without adjustment for any differences among regions, the HRR in the 90th percentile of spending spent 42 percent more per Medicare beneficiary each month than the HRR in the 10th percentile. Analyses of commercial insurance data confirm the presence of similar spending variation (a 36-42 percent difference between the 90th and 10th percentiles of HRR-level spending) for all geographic units (HSA, HRR, and metropolitan CBSA), with greater variation at the smaller, HSA level. A separate analysis of Medicare Advantage (Medicare Part C), as well as an estimate of total health care spending in the United States, likewise found remarkable regional differences between the highest- and lowest-spending quintiles at the HRR level, with 90th/10th percentile ratios of 1.36 and 1.50, respectively.

Variation can be found at all geographic levels. Medicare spending, however, adjusted for regional differences in age, sex, and health status, is correlated only weakly with spending among the privately insured population (correlations of 0.08-0.11) at the HRR level. In other words, areas that are high spenders in Medicare are not necessarily high spenders in the commercial market and vice versa.

All of the subcontractors examined variation in the utilization of prescription drugs; imaging procedures; and inpatient, outpatient, and

---

[3]The committee's conclusions are numbered according to the chapter of the main text in which they appear.

emergency department care. The Acumen Medicare analysis additionally evaluated variation in post-acute care services. The ratios of the 90th/10th percentiles of risk-adjusted utilization (measured as counts) point to the presence of regional variation across a number and variety of health care services within the Medicare and commercial payer populations.

The committee determined geographic variation to be a true signal rather than a result of random noise, as regional differences in health care spending and utilization persist over time. The subcontractor analyses demonstrate that growth rates of Medicare spending and utilization are consistent over time for high- and low-cost regions in the country. In other words, regions that were high- (or low-) cost in 1992 remained high- (or low-) cost in 2010. Further, area-level Medicare and commercial spending and utilization are highly correlated from one year to the next between 1992 and 2010, suggesting that geographic variation arises from systematic differences rather than randomness.

Conclusion 2.2. Variation in spending in the commercial insurance market is due mainly to differences in price markups by providers rather than to differences in the utilization of health care services.

Variation in health care spending reflects variation in both price and utilization (quantity of services). "Price" is the amount paid by insurers and beneficiaries to a provider per unit of health care services. Whereas CMS traditionally sets a uniform national base price, adjusting for the differences in input prices across geographic areas and for certain other factors, commercial prices are set through negotiations between providers and payers. Because negotiating power (on both sides) varies across areas, the variation in prices received by providers is substantially larger in the commercial sector than in Medicare.

Analyses conducted for this study support the results in the existing literature, which indicate that adjusting for regional differences in input prices has little effect on observed variation in Medicare spending. In the commercial market, however, regional differences in prices paid by insurers to providers, rather than utilization of health care, influence much of the overall regional variation in spending. Harvard's analysis of commercial MarketScan data disaggregated unit price into its subcomponents and examined variation in input prices and markups (defined as the difference between input and transaction "output" prices). Harvard reports that 70 percent of variation in total commercial spending is attributable to price markups, most likely reflecting the varying market power of providers across HRRs. Although utilization of various services, particularly rates of inpatient admissions and emergency department visits, does contribute to regional differences in spending, it has a notably smaller influence than price markups (see the related discussion in Chapter 2).

Conclusion 2.3. The committee's empirical analysis revealed that after accounting for differences in age, sex, and health status, geographic variation is not further explained by other beneficiary demographic factors, insurance plan factors, or market-level characteristics. In fact, after controlling for all factors measurable within the data used for this analysis, a large amount of variation remains unexplained.

A number of factors contribute to geographic variation, and while many of these factors traditionally have been classified as "acceptable" or "unacceptable," some sources of variation are ambiguous and do not fall neatly into either category. The committee's analyses generally adjusted for acceptable variation, which results from factors beyond the control of the health care system in a region. To quantify these effects, the subcontractors conducted multiple regression analyses, adjusting for various "clusters" or groups of predictors. The results indicate that adjusting for age and sex (Cluster 1) has a negligible effect on geographic variation in Medicare spending. Beneficiary health status (Cluster 2), when measured using diagnoses recorded on claims, substantially reduces variation between high- and low-spending regions across both the Medicare and commercial payer sectors. This reduction in unexplained geographic variation is illustrated in Figure S-1. As indicated by the narrowed distribution of the 90th/10th percentile ratios (1.44 to 1.23) in the lower histogram, a greater number of HRRs (weighted by beneficiary months) fall in the middle range of Medicare spending after adjustment for age, sex, and health status.

As discussed in Chapter 2, other demographic factors, such as race, income, insurance and employer characteristics, and market factors, have a trivial effect on reducing variation once beneficiary health status is included in the model. Even after adjusting for all predictors measurable within the data used for this study and supported by the literature, a substantial amount of variation remains unexplained. PHE's analysis of variation in total, input-price-adjusted health care spending attributable to known predictors reveals a pattern similar to that of Medicare- and commercial-only spending.

The subcontractors' analyses do not distinguish between "acceptable" and "unacceptable" sources of variation. The residual unexplained variation unaccounted for here may have a causal connection with unobservable factors such as patient preferences, unmeasured regional differences in health status, market characteristics, or discretionary provision of inefficient care. However, the robust presence of variation, even with adjust-

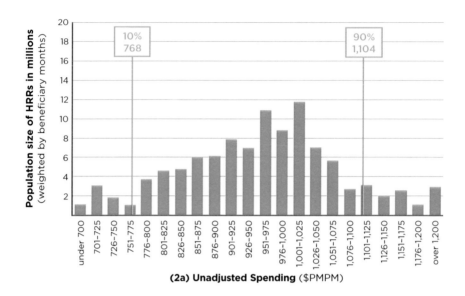

(2a) Unadjusted Spending ($PMPM)

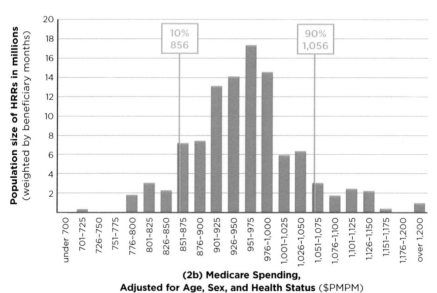

**(2b) Medicare Spending,
Adjusted for Age, Sex, and Health Status** ($PMPM)

FIGURE S-1 Number of Medicare beneficiaries in hospital referral regions (HRRs) in 22 categories of monthly per capita spending, with input-price adjustment alone (2a—top) and with input-price adjustment plus adjustment for age, sex, and health status (2b—bottom).

NOTE: Medicare spending in both 2a and 2b have been adjusted for regional difference in input price. PMPM = per patient per month.

SOURCE: Developed by the committee and IOM staff based on data from Acumen Medicare analysis.

ment for more and more "acceptable" factors, creates a presumption that inefficiency may be one of the potential causes of variation.

> *Conclusion 2.4. Variation in total Medicare spending across geographic areas is driven largely by variation in the utilization of post-acute care services, and to a lesser extent by variation in the utilization of acute care services.*

To determine the extent to which variation in particular health care services contributes to total variation in Medicare spending, the committee disaggregated price-standardized, risk-adjusted Medicare spending into seven types of services: (1) acute (inpatient) care, (2) post-acute care, (3) prescription drugs, (4) diagnostics, (5) procedures, (6) emergency department visits, and (7) other. The subcontractors' analyses suggest that utilization of post-acute care services is a key driver of HRR-level variation in Medicare spending, with most of the remaining variation stemming from the use of acute (inpatient) care services.

As Table S-1 indicates, if there were no variation in post-acute care spending, the variation in total Medicare spending across HRRs would fall

TABLE S-1
Proportion of Variance Attributable to Each Medicare Service Category

	Adjusted Total Medicare Spending	
	Remaining Variance	Reduction in Variance (%)*
Variation in Total Medicare Spending	6,974	—
If No Variation in Post-Acute Care Only	1,864	73
If No Variation in Acute Care Only	5,085	27
If No Variation in Either Post-Acute or Acute	780	89
If No Variation in Prescription Drugs	6,374	9
If No Variation in Diagnostic Tests	5,986	14
If No Variation in Procedures	6,020	14
If No Variation in Emergency Department Visits/Ambulance Use	6,972	0
If No Variation in Other	6,882	1

NOTE: Total Medicare spending and each component are input-price- and risk-adjusted using a diagnostic-based measure of risk (CMS—hierarchical condition categories [HCCs]). Each row shows the reduction in variance from eliminating only the variation in that service, with the exception of the acute and post-acute care rows.

*The individual reductions sum to more than 100 percent because of covariance terms.

SOURCE: Committee analysis of Medicare data.

by 73 percent. If there were no variation in acute care spending, but the variation in post-acute care spending were unchanged, the variation in total spending would fall by 27 percent. Finally, if there were no variation in either acute or post-acute care spending, variation in total spending would fall by 89 percent. Thus, the remaining services shown (e.g., diagnostic, which includes outpatient physician services; emergency room/ambulance service; prescription drugs) play only a small role in variation in Medicare spending.

Research and Data Limitations

The committee's commissioned analyses evaluated quality of care using individual measures and the following nationally established composite quality indicators: a Prevention Quality Indicator (PQI), which measures the quality of ambulatory care; an Inpatient Quality Composite Indicator (IQI), which measures quality in an inpatient hospital setting; a Patient Safety Indicator (PSI), which measures the quality of inpatient care as it relates to preventable complications; and a Pediatric Quality Indicator (PDI), which reflects the quality of care among the pediatric population. Although these national quality indicators represent the "current state of the art in assessing the health care system as a whole," performance measures based on administrative data have a number of limitations. Because of these limitations in measurement of quality composites and underlying data, this report does not quantify the amount of geographic variation in health care quality as it does for spending and utilization.

As noted earlier, a number of methodological challenges and a lack of data precluded thorough analyses of geographic variation among the Medicaid and uninsured populations. Although CMS has in recent years attempted to improve and simplify the process of obtaining historical data, significant operational, procedural, and financial barriers remain. Congress could help remove these barriers by supporting CMS's efforts to expand the availability of Medicare and Medicaid data for research purposes. It would be particularly valuable if CMS were to release the previously unavailable or limited Medicare Part C and D databases that it maintains.

More research on health care outcomes and quality is needed, particularly in commercially insured populations. Many nationally established composite measures of quality are designed to measure process and outcomes in the Medicare population and are not necessarily applicable to privately insured beneficiaries. Further research is needed in this area, and this work would benefit from the availability of a national-level all-payer database. Moreover, combined use of Medicare and private administrative or claims data would allow for more accurate measurement of provider performance and quality of care.

RECOMMENDATION 1: Congress should encourage the Centers for Medicare & Medicaid Services (CMS), and provide the necessary resources, to make accessing Medicare and Medicaid data easier for research purposes. CMS should collaborate with private insurers to collect, integrate, and analyze standardized data on spending, as well as clinical and behavioral health outcomes, to enable more extensive comparisons of payments and quality and evaluation of value-based payment models across payers.

EVALUATION OF THE USE OF A GEOGRAPHIC VALUE INDEX

An important part of the committee's statement of task and research framework focuses on "whether Medicare payment systems should be modified to provide incentives for high-value, high-quality, evidence-based, patient-centered care through adoption of a value index (based on measures of quality and cost) that would adjust payments on a geographic area basis." To create a research framework that would generate useful information for policy makers, the committee needed to understand the dimensions of the geographically based value index described in its statement of task.

In general, a value index is a relative measure of value—for example, a measure of improvement in patient-centered clinical health outcomes per unit of resources used in one area relative to the national average. The committee defined health care value as the equivalent of net benefit: the amount by which overall health benefit and/or well-being produced by care exceeds (or falls short of) the costs of producing it. Those costs should incorporate the opportunity costs of resources used to produce medical services. But because opportunity costs seldom are observed directly, the committee defined "costs" for purposes of this study as Medicare or other payer spending for goods and services. These observed costs are based on payment formulas that bear some relation to opportunity costs, but they could differ considerably. Note also that economic efficiency reflects not only obtaining the most utility from a given set of inputs, but also investing the proper amount of inputs in a given activity relative to others. Thus, assessing value in health care requires a measure of society's and/or an individual's willingness to pay for certain services relative to others.

Assessing the value of health care goods and services is challenging, requiring appropriate measures of health benefits, well-being, and cost. To operationalize the committee's definition of value, health benefit must be valued in a consistent fashion, typically using either dollars or quality-adjusted life years. Cost is valued in dollars. Because a health care system is designed to promote health through the provision of health care services, taking into account the system's fiscal sustainability, health outcomes are a logical choice for assessing the overall health benefit or well-being attributable to health care. However, it is rarely straightforward to ascertain the contribution of an individual health care service to a specific health outcome, particularly in the management of chronic conditions.

Value Indexes

Value indexes can take specific forms and serve many purposes. In health care, they can be used to adjust hospital or provider reimbursement rates based on measures of relative performance. For example, CMS's hospital value-based purchasing program and physician payment modifier (authorized under Sections 3001 and 3007 of the ACA, respectively) adjust hospital and provider payments according to observed hospital and individual provider performance compared with national averages. Health benefit and well-being are, of course, affected by many factors other than the provision of health care services, such as individual behavior, biology, and genetics. If a value index influences health care payments, it is important that related measures of health outcomes be attributable to specific health care interventions. Therefore, clinical health outcomes (i.e., the health status of a patient resulting from health care) may be a preferred measure of health benefit or well-being.

As described above, this report focuses primarily on a geographically based value index. Section 1159 of the Affordable Health Care for America Act (H.R. 3962), on which the committee's charge is based, asked the IOM to consider different value indexes, including a value index that would adjust provider payments based on regional composite measures of quality and cost. Thus, the committee limited its evaluation of a "geographically based value index" to a relative ratio that uses area-level composite measures of clinical health outcomes and cost to adjust individual hospital and provider payments under Medicare Parts A and B ("a geographic value index").[4]

Conclusion 3.1. A geographically based value index is unlikely to promote more efficient behaviors among individual providers and thus is unlikely to improve the overall value of health care.

Health care decision making generally occurs at the level of the individual practitioner or organization (e.g., hospital or physician group), not at the level of a geographic region. A geographic value index is not designed

---

[4]Note that such an index differs from CMS's hospital value-based purchasing program and physician payment modifier, as described above.

to target any level of actual decision making. Rather, it treats all providers in an area alike, assuming that area-level payment modifications will incentivize the various decision makers within an area to coordinate care and improve efficiencies across the area. However, two practical considerations suggest otherwise. First, collaboration among competing providers, absent clinical and financial integration, may raise antitrust issues. Second, payment modifications that target large areas do not always link individual physician behaviors to spending increases or decreases.

Although setting provider payments by geographic region is more targeted than the current sustainable growth rate (SGR) system, it raises similar practical concerns. In most cases, geographic regions (HRR, metropolitan CBSA) large enough to have stable year-to-year spending are too large for any individual provider to have enough influence over total expenditures to alter provider behavior patterns. When a single delivery system dominates in an area, payment policies targeting geographically based government units are functionally equivalent to targeting the relevant decision-making unit. In other cases, health care payment systems may appropriately target regional or community-based "collaboratives." However, because such collaboratives often vary in size and structure and are not necessarily tied to central budgets within their communities, they may or may not comport with traditional geographic units.

Conclusion 3.2. Substantial variation in spending and utilization remains as units of analysis get progressively smaller.

A geographic value index for Medicare would have to generate hospital and provider payments perceived as fair. But area-level payments are fair only under certain conditions. First, all hospitals and providers within an area must be equally deserving of reward (or penalty), implying that they behave similarly. Second, assuming all providers are behaving similarly, performance levels in high-value areas must be achievable in low-value areas through elimination of inefficiencies. In other words, differences in measured value between low- and high-spending areas cannot include differences stemming from underlying health status and other acceptable sources of variation.

Spending Variation at Different Levels

Starting with HRRs, the committee examined amounts of variation within progressively smaller units of analysis (HSA, hospital, practice, and individual provider levels).

Spending Variation at the Hospital Service Area Level Within Hospital Referral Regions

The empirical analyses conducted for this study reveal evidence of substantial geographic variation in Medicare spending at the HSA level within HRR regions. As one measure of variability within an HRR, the committee examined the ratio of the highest-Medicare-spending to the lowest-Medicare-spending HSA within each HRR.[5] In the 76 HRRs with the highest ratios (those above the 75th percentile), the highest-spending HSA within each HRR spends at least 36 percent more per Medicare beneficiary than the lowest-spending HSA within that HRR. The separate analysis by PHE found that approximately 40 to 70 percent of variation in spending and utilization remained after controlling for HRR characteristics. Collectively, these findings demonstrate considerable variation in spending and utilization that can be explained not by HRR-level factors but by factors at the smaller, HSA geographic level or even below that level, within HSAs.

Spending Variation at the Hospital Level Within Hospital Referral Regions

Hospitals within the same HRR vary substantially in their resource use, as can be seen from the committee's analysis of Dartmouth data on variation in hospital spending for cohorts of patients treated for three major conditions—stroke, hip fracture, and heart attack.[6] This variation among hospitals exists in both lower- and higher-spending HRRs, meaning there are high-spending hospitals in low-spending regions and low-spending hospitals in high-spending regions, as illustrated in Figure S-2.

Spending Variation Within Provider Practices

The committee could not examine variation below the hospital level (i.e., at the provider level) in its analyses of Medicare data because of privacy concerns. However, supplementary analyses of data from Blue Cross Blue Shield of Massachusetts indicate that variation among specialists working in the same group practice is as great as that among specialists across the entire state.

---

[5] This analysis was limited to HRRs with three or more HSAs.

[6] This analysis was limited to HRRs containing four or more hospitals with data on spending for a given condition.

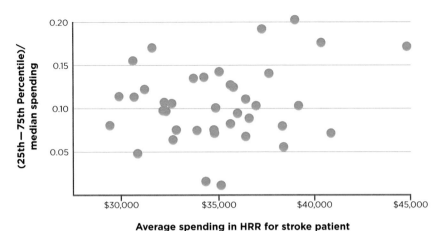

FIGURE S-2 Variation in price- and risk-adjusted Medicare spending for stroke in a hospital referral region.
SOURCE: Committee analysis of unpublished Dartmouth data.

Spending Variation at the Individual Provider Level Across Clinical Conditions

Even individual physician performance varies across different performance measures. A study by Partners Healthcare found substantial variation in utilization and quality of health care services even within a single practice group comprising six primary care physicians. The study analyzed nine distinct quality measures applied to diabetes, cholesterol, and hypertension control; ordering of radiology tests and generic prescriptions; and rates of admissions and emergency department visits. No single physician scored consistently high or low across all measures; instead, each was above average for some and below average for others. These data demonstrate the difficulty of using composite measures to classify individual physicians as high- or low-value providers.

Since providers within a region do not behave similarly, use of a geographic value index would raise a fairness issue, as low-value providers would be rewarded simply for practicing in areas that are on average high-value (the reverse would also be true). As a result, area-level performance calculations would likely mischaracterize the actual value of services delivered by many providers and hospitals, resulting in unfair payments.

Conclusion 3.3. Quality across conditions and treatments varies widely within HRRs; spending and utilization across conditions are moderately correlated within HRRs.

Although claims-based quality measures are sparse in some specialized clinical areas, they are plentiful and robust in others. Because a geographic value index calculates a composite quality score for a region, many providers in an area will be evaluated on measures not applicable to their own practices. Therefore, for a geographic value index to generate fair reimbursement rates, data would at a minimum have to indicate that performance across a wide range of quality measures was relatively consistent within an area.

The Medicare and Harvard analyses found that areas with high scores on some quality measures do not necessarily have high scores on others, particularly if the measures relate to conditions treated by different types of specialists. In the Medicare analyses, pairwise correlations between 18 condition-specific quality indicators showed that approximately 38 percent of quality measure pairs are negatively correlated with each other, 40 percent have correlation coefficients between 0 and 0.19, and only one-fifth have correlation coefficients above 0.20. Collectively, these findings suggest that an area in which providers deliver high-value treatment for one condition may well contain providers who deliver low-value treatment for other conditions. In other words, the findings confirm that provider performance is not homogeneous within an area.

Within an HRR, moreover, spending and utilization measures across conditions are more highly correlated than quality measures. Nonetheless, an HRR that uses many services to treat a given condition (e.g., prostate cancer) does not necessarily use many services to treat another (e.g., low back pain).

Conclusion 3.4. HRR-level quality is not consistently related to spending or utilization in Medicare or the commercial sector.

Use of a geographic value index would require that area-level performance be observable in reliable relationships between health care resource use and health care quality. Thus, assuming that composite measures of health care spending and health outcomes are used to measure value, the case for an area-wide payment adjuster is stronger if a payment change has consistent effects on the quality measures making up the composites.

The committee's commissioned analyses did not reveal a consistent relationship between condition-specific utilization and condition-specific quality measures in the Medicare population. Positive correlations between utilization and quality measures varied from 0.005 for radiation therapy for breast cancer to 0.085 for disease-modifying antirheumatic drugs dispensed for arthritis (0.085). Negative correlations between utilization and quality measures ranged from −0.012 to −0.048. Similarly, Harvard's MarketScan analysis found both positive and negative correlations between spending and quality, depending on the specific measure tested.

In sum, acknowledging the limitations and challenges to interpretation of the quality analyses, overall the committee found no evidence of reliable associations between disease- or condition-specific measures of utilization and disease- or condition-specific measures of quality. Findings from the committee's commissioned empirical analyses are consistent with those of a recent systematic review by Hussey et al.,[7] demonstrating an inconsistent relationship between health care quality and cost. As a result, a geographic value index employing these measures could affect some health outcomes negatively and others positively.

> **RECOMMENDATION 2: Congress should not adopt a geographically based value index for Medicare. Because geographic units are not where most health care decisions are made, a geographic value index would be a poorly targeted mechanism for encouraging value improvement. Adjusting payments geographically, based on any aggregate or composite measure of spending or quality, would unfairly reward low-value providers in high-value regions and punish high-value providers in low-value regions.**

PAYMENT AND ORGANIZATIONAL REFORMS TO IMPROVE VALUE

Those who characterize the U.S. health care system as highly inefficient cite evidence of underuse, overuse, and misuse of medical services throughout the health care delivery system. A number of factors contribute to inefficiency, including information asymmetries, fragmentation in the organization and delivery of health care services, and the widespread prevalence of fee-for-service reimbursement. The statement of task for this study asked the committee to recommend payment reforms that would promote the delivery of high-value care while taking into consideration the ACA and related changes already under way.

The delivery of health care involves myriad decisions by a wide range of decision makers, including solo practitioners, single-specialty group practices, multiple-specialty group practices, hospitals, health care systems, and in some cases community-based multistakeholder collaboratives. The committee's research illustrates how variation in spending and quality exists in progressively smaller units, down to the hospital, single-specialty group practice, and even individual physician levels, suggesting that opportunities

---

[7]Hussey, P. S., S. Wertheimer, and A. Mehrotra. 2013. The association between health care quality and cost: A systematic review. *Annals of Internal Medicine* 158(1):27-34.

for value improvement exist at all levels of health care decision making. Depending on the organizational setting and degree of clinical integration, different decision makers have varying abilities to maximize efficiencies and improve value.

> RECOMMENDATION 3: To improve value, the Centers for Medicare & Medicaid Services (CMS) should continue to test payment reforms that incentivize the clinical and financial integration of health care delivery systems and thereby encourage their (1) coordination of care among individual providers, (2) real-time sharing of data and tracking of service use and health outcomes, (3) receipt and distribution of provider payments, and (4) assumption of some or all of the risk of managing the care continuum for their populations. Further, CMS should pilot programs that allow beneficiaries to share in the savings due to higher-value care.

To improve value, payment reforms need to create incentives for behavioral change at the locus of care (provider and patient). Therefore, payment should target decision-making units, whether they be at the level of individual providers, hospitals, health care systems, or stakeholder collaboratives. A growing body of evidence leads to the conclusion that clinical and financial integration best positions health care systems to manage the continuum of care for their complex populations efficiently. Clinical integration denotes a minimum level of coordination and alignment of goals among providers (physicians, hospitals, and other practitioners) caring for a population. In clinically integrated environments, providers share clinical data, agree on plans of care, and collaborate to achieve favorable patient-centered outcomes. Hence, at minimum, they must foster care coordination among individual providers, as well as share data and track service use and outcomes to measure progress. Financial integration often hastens clinical integration. Financially integrated health care systems have the capability to receive payments and distribute them to individual care providers. Doing so allows health care systems to align financial incentives among providers within organizations.

However, financial integration is not a unitary goal; historically, financially integrated health care organizations lacking management, infrastructure, and processes for coordinating care (i.e., clinical integration) generally have not succeeded in substantially lowering costs or improving care quality. Clinical and financial integration may in some markets increase provider concentration, enabling providers in those markets to charge commercial carriers higher prices. Antitrust enforcement often raises a difficult trade-off between production efficiencies and market power, and health care is no exception. Nonetheless, greater value clearly requires greater coordination among providers.

Therefore, payers can promote value through payment and organizational reforms that foster the above elements of clinical and financial integration. In fact, many payment reforms included in the ACA and tested in the commercial market (e.g., value-based purchasing, bundled payment, accountable care organizations, patient-centered medical home models, and dual-eligible care integration demonstrations) do just that. Table S-2 provides a brief description of selected payment reforms. Because these reforms are relatively new, evidence on their influence on value is limited. Early provider reaction has been positive, as reflected in the larger-than-anticipated number of organizations contracting with CMS to join pilot programs. However, the U.S. health care delivery system encompasses a diverse array of provider organizational relationships, which vary in size, level of integration (both clinical and financial), and ability/willingness to assume financial risk. Therefore, it is advisable for CMS to test payment

TABLE S-2
Payment Reforms Included in the Patient Protection and Affordable Care Act

Payment Reform	Description
Value-based purchasing	Under a value-based purchasing program, providers—such as hospitals, medical groups, and nursing homes—receive greater reimbursement if they attain a high level of performance on quality or cost measures or improve their performance on such measures by a sufficient degree.
Bundled payment	Under bundled payment, a payer makes a single payment for all services (a bundle) provided during an episode of care.
Accountable care organizations (ACOs)	The ACO is a health care delivery and financing model currently being tested by the Centers for Medicare & Medicaid Services (CMS) and commercial insurers. ACO reforms target organized provider organizations and networks that assume responsibility for the quality, cost, and overall care of their patient populations.
Patient-centered medical home (PCMH)	The PCMH is a health care delivery model that organizes the care continuum around a practitioner team with the primary care provider at the center, helping patients coordinate care and manage chronic conditions. The PCMH also generally incorporates evidence-based medicine and quality improvement activities.
Dual-eligible care integration	CMS has provided grants to allow states to undertake care integration initiatives for dual-eligible populations. One goal of the demonstrations is to determine which care integration and payment models are most effective in improving the quality and efficiency of care for this heterogeneous population.

models that are compatible with less as well as more clinically integrated providers to see how reforms impact the value of care in different settings.

Finally, patients are also health care decision makers, and can be encouraged through alternative cost-sharing arrangements to share in the savings derived from higher-value care. Introducing value-based cost sharing into a health care system may encourage patients to choose high-value providers and/or higher-value care options. However, increasing cost sharing has been shown to decrease utilization of both effective and ineffective services; thus, more information is needed on how best to tailor a program to encourage the selection of higher-value care options. To this end, CMS could pilot programs aimed at aligning patient cost-sharing arrangements with value.

> **RECOMMENDATION 4: During the transition to new payment models, the Centers for Medicare & Medicaid Services (CMS) should conduct ongoing evaluations of the impact on value of the reforms included in Recommendation 3 by measuring Medicare spending and beneficiaries' clinical health outcomes. CMS should use the results of these evaluations to iteratively improve these payment models. CMS should also monitor how these reforms impact Medicare beneficiaries' access to medical care.**

By creating the Center for Medicare and Medicaid Innovation, the ACA generated a thousand pilot demonstrations of value-based payment models. It is too early to know which of these models will prove to control health care costs and improve quality. Evidence supporting the effectiveness of new payment models such as value-based purchasing, patient-centered medical homes, bundled payment, and accountable care organizations in controlling costs and improving health outcomes is limited. Given that these models are still in the early stages of development, however, it is critical that CMS continue to evaluate them and use the results to refine their design.

Further, as reforms transition from pilot demonstrations to broader programs, CMS will need to monitor Medicare beneficiaries' access to care. Value-based payment reforms are designed to reward efficient providers of care and drive inefficient providers to improve care processes. Some providers/health systems will flourish with these new incentives; others will struggle and may fail. It is also likely that local market factors (e.g., population demographics, provider competition) will influence providers' abilities to handle new payments, so models suited for some areas will face greater challenges in others. While some disruption to the current system is inevitable and even warranted, it is critical that Medicare beneficiaries' access to care not be diminished.

RECOMMENDATION 5: If evaluations of specific payment reforms demonstrate increased value, Congress should give the Centers for Medicare & Medicaid Services the flexibility to accelerate the transition from traditional Medicare to new payment models.

Translating new payment models to national policy will be a challenge. If new payment models were mandated before a majority of health care providers had developed the required infrastructure, many organizational failures (e.g., bankruptcies) might result, negatively affecting Medicare beneficiaries' access to care. Similarly, provider organizations will voluntarily accept new payment models only if they believe payments will cover their investment in the infrastructure required to achieve efficiencies, as well as generate bonuses or shared savings. Particularly in the beginning, therefore, instead of employing a mandatory approach, Congress might direct CMS to accelerate the adoption of payment reforms by authorizing differential payment updates for new payment models and traditional Medicare. It should also be noted that providers serving disproportionately low-income populations may face especially difficult challenges in accessing the necessary resources, and may require additional funding to build the organizational capacity to transition to the new payment models.

Additionally, Congress should give CMS the flexibility to experiment with the mix of payment mechanisms, rates, and performance metrics that will align provider incentives with high-value care. For example, CMS might test a blended payment model for patient-centered medical homes that combines fee-for-service payments, per-member-per-month care coordination fees, and bonuses for meeting quality and efficiency metrics (e.g., generic prescribing, reduced emergency room use, better management of selected chronic conditions). While evaluations are ongoing, CMS should be allowed to alter the levels and payment rates within models to determine those that are most effective.

1

Introduction and Overview

In 2009, following negotiations over the Patient Protection and Affordable Care Act (ACA),[1] a group of members of the House of Representatives known as the Quality Care Coalition asked Secretary of Health and Human Services (HHS) Kathleen Sebelius to sponsor two Institute of Medicine (IOM) studies focused on geographic payments under Medicare, independent of final health care reform legislation (Sebelius, 2010). The first study evaluated the accuracy of Medicare's geographic adjustment factors, which alter physician and hospital payment rates based on geographically based input prices. The IOM released two reports based on that first study—*Geographic Adjustment in Medicare Payment—Phase 1: Improving Accuracy* and *Geographic Adjustment in Medicare Payment—Phase II: Implications for Access, Quality, and Efficiency*—in 2011 and 2012, respectively (IOM, 2011, 2012b).

For the second study, documented in the present report, the Centers for Medicare & Medicaid Services (CMS) contracted with the IOM to conduct a 3-year consensus study to investigate geographic variation in health care spending and quality and to analyze Medicare payment polices that could encourage high-value care, including the adoption of a geographically based value index. This index would in principle account for both the health benefit obtained from health care services delivered and the cost of those services, as discussed later in this report. Deputy Director Jonathan Blum described CMS's motivation for commissioning the study as an effort "to

---

[1] Patient Protection and Affordable Care Act, Public Law 111-148, 111th Cong., 2nd sess., (March 23, 2010).

build more consensus about ... the reasons, the causes, and the impacts for health care spending variation—to help [CMS] develop policies to address those variations."[2]

Although the IOM has never published a report focused on geographic variation in health care spending and quality, the topic is a familiar one. Many IOM consensus reports and workshop summaries provide findings, conclusions, and recommendations on issues related to geographic variation, such as improving health care quality (IOM, 2001, 2002, 2003, 2006a), reducing health care spending (IOM, 2010a; NRC, 2010), and improving value within the U.S. health care system (IOM, 2006b, 2010b, 2012b). The committee formed to conduct the present study drew on this prior work for conceptual and methodological insight.

SPENDING AND HEALTH CARE QUALITY IN THE UNITED STATES

There is broad consensus that U.S. health care expenditures have been growing at an unsustainable rate. In 2011, total U.S. health care expenditures amounted to $2.7 trillion, or 17.9 percent of national gross domestic product (GDP), substantially more than was spent by other developed countries (CMS, 2013; Kaiser Family Foundation, 2012). The Congressional Budget Office (CBO) projects that federal health care spending will total $7.94 trillion between 2014 and 2023 (ModernHealthcare.com, 2013). At current expenditure rates, moreover, the Medicare Hospital Insurance Trust Fund (which covers the cost of Medicare Part A hospital insurance benefits for Medicare beneficiaries) will be insolvent by the mid-2020s (Social Security and Medicare Boards of Trustees, 2008). Growing health care expenditures also strain state budgets (National Governors Association and National Association of State Budget Officers, 2012; The Pew Center on the States, 2012) and threaten the well-being of individuals and families (Schoen et al., 2011; World Bank, 2012).

Despite the tremendous resources dedicated to health care, health care quality in the United States remains inconsistent. Significant advances in biomedical sciences, medicine, and public health have contributed to better individual and population health, including increased life expectancy and state-of-the-art cancer treatment (Docteur and Berenson, 2009). However, systematic underuse, misuse, and overuse of medical services throughout the U.S. health care system contribute to decreased quality of patient care (IOM, 1999). For example, approximately one in seven Medicare beneficiaries experiences an adverse event during a hospital stay, resulting in 15,000

---

[2]2010 (November 9). Speech before the Committee on Geographic Variation in Health Care Spending and Promotion of High-Value Care. Washington, DC: National Academy of Sciences.

avoidable deaths each month (Levinson, 2010). The CBO estimates that medical negligence contributes to 181,000 severe medical injuries each year (CBO, 2008). In 2009, Medicare paid an estimated $4.4 billion to care for patients who had been harmed in the hospital and $26 billion for hospital readmissions. Even as they threaten the welfare of patients, inefficiencies within the health care system divert limited resources from other national priorities, such as education, infrastructure, and debt reduction.

MEDICARE PAYMENT POLICY REFORM AND GEOGRAPHIC VARIATION IN SPENDING AND QUALITY

For more than three decades, experts at the Dartmouth Institute for Health Policy and Clinical Practice ("Dartmouth") have documented significant variation in Medicare spending and quality across geographic regions,[3] producing a series of maps that have become known as the *Dartmouth Atlas of Health Care* (Dartmouth Institute for Health Policy and Clinical Practice, 2013; Wennberg and Cooper, 1999). From this seminal body of work, a finding emerged that health care spending and rates of utilization of specific services varied widely but did not appear to be consistently related to health outcomes or patient satisfaction among Medicare beneficiaries (Baicker and Chandra, 2004; Fisher et al., 2003a,b; MedPAC, 2009, 2011; Zhang et al., 2010).

A central question in the debate about geographic variation is the following: Should Medicare's policy for paying health care providers be modified in light of the possibility that Medicare beneficiaries in high-spending areas do not experience better health outcomes? In fact, some legislators have asked whether cutting Medicare payment rates to high-cost areas might save money without adversely affecting health care quality for beneficiaries. The authors of one study assert that Medicare spending would drop by as much as 29 percent if practices of low-cost, high-quality regions were adopted nationwide, while health care for Medicare beneficiaries would significantly improve (Wennberg et al., 2002). Moreover, some argue that Medicare's traditional fee-for-service reimbursement system is a major driver of both variation and waste because it rewards providers based on the volume and intensity rather than the value of services delivered. For instance, congressional representatives in areas generally associated with high-quality, low-cost health care argue that highly efficient hospitals and providers are penalized under the current payment system.[4]

Based on these observations, some lawmakers have proposed that

---

[3]Hospital referral regions (HRRs) and hospital service areas (HSAs); see Chapter 2, Box 2-1, for definitions.

[4]Personal communication, Michael Kitchell, Iowa Medical Society, January 7, 2011.

Medicare should adjust physician reimbursement rates based on regional performance to encourage more uniform performance of the health care system for Medicare beneficiaries across hospital markets.[5,6,7] Proponents of a geographic value index theorize that such regional payment adjustments would encourage all hospitals and providers within an area to coordinate care, leading to better system efficiencies across the region.[8,9]

Other health care experts counter that supporters of the above policy proposal conflate the issue of improving value with that of reducing geographic variation. They point out that some variation in health care spending is to be expected in an efficient health care system, reflecting anticipated differences in consumption of health care services by individual patients. They argue that reducing geographic variation is desirable only to the extent that measured variation represents inefficiencies in the health care system. This concept is explored further in Chapter 2.

Still other health care experts argue that regionally based payments are inherently unfair and would fail to create market incentives necessary to promote high-value, patient-centered care. Region-level measures of variation mask variation within regions. Specifically, such finer-grained variation means provider payments based on regional area performance would reward inefficient providers in low-cost regions and punish more efficient providers in high-cost regions (MedPAC, 2007). Given the public and private resources at stake and the need for improved health care quality, lawmakers and health care experts demanded additional research and expert opinion to inform the debate on geographic variation. Examples of these arguments, presented at the public workshops held for this study, are offered later in this chapter.

STUDY CHARGE AND SCOPE

To conduct this study, the IOM convened the Committee on Geographic Variation in Health Care Spending and Promotion of High-Value Care, whose 19 members included experts in health economics, statistics, health care financing, value-based health care purchasing, health services research, health law, and health disparities. The committee's statement of

---

[5]Medicare Payment Improvement Act of 2009, S. 1249, 111th Cong., 1st sess. (June 12, 2009).

[6]Medicare Payment Improvement Act of 2009, H.R. 2844, 111th Cong., 1st sess. (June 15, 2009).

[7]It should be noted that Dartmouth researchers do not recommend the use of a geographically based value index (Skinner et al., 2010).

[8]Personal communication, Michael Richards, Gundersen Lutheran Health Services, January 17, 2011.

[9]U.S. Congress, Senate. 2009. Health Care Reform. 111th Cong. (July 30, 2009).

task (see Box 1-1) draws on language in earlier federal health care reform legislation[10] and includes the following three tasks[11]:

1. to independently evaluate geographic variation in health care spending levels and growth among Medicare, Medicaid, privately insured, and uninsured populations in the United States;
2. to make recommendations for changes in Medicare Part A, B, and C payments, considering findings from task 1, as well as changes to Medicare payment systems under the ACA; and
3. to address whether Medicare payments for physicians and hospitals should incorporate a value index that would modify the payments based on geographic-area performance.

STUDY METHODS

This section describes the methods used to conduct this study. The first step was to formulate an operational definition of value in health care. Then, to evaluate geographic variation in health care costs and quality and thereby value, the committee commissioned an extensive body of new statistical analyses and four papers from subject-matter experts and held two public workshops to complement its review of the existing literature.

Definition of Value

To respond to its statement of task, the committee identified two basic questions:

1. What is known about geographic variation in health care spending, utilization, and quality?
2. Should geographically based measures of value be used to adjust Medicare fee-for-service hospital and provider reimbursement rates in a geographic region?

Before seeking to answer these questions, the committee needed to adopt an operational definition of "value." In health care, the term "value" is used widely but imprecisely and with very different meanings. A common thread is the notion of efficiency, as in health services or health outcomes achieved per unit costs, where outcomes encompass a variety of health di-

---

[10]The Affordable Health Care for America Act, H.R. 3962, 111th Cong., 1st sess. (October 29, 2009).

[11]Preservation of Access to Care for Medicare Beneficiaries and Pension Relief Act of 2010, Public Law 111-192, 111th Cong., 2nd sess. (June 25, 2010).

BOX 1-1
Statement of Task

An ad hoc committee will conduct a study on geographic variation in intensity, cost, and growth of health care services and in per capita health care spending among the Medicare, Medicaid, privately insured, and un-insured U.S. populations as proposed in Section 1159 of the Affordable Health Care for America Act (H.R. 3962) in 2009, and commissioned by the Secretary, U.S. Department of Health and Human Services, in 2010.

The committee will commission relevant new analyses and will evaluate and review factors such as:

- Variation in areas of different sizes;
- Input prices; health status; practice patterns; access to medical services; supply of medical services; socioeconomic factors, including race, ethnicity, gender, age, income and educational status; and provider and payment organizations;
- Patient access to care, insurance status, distribution of health care resources, health care outcomes and quality;
- Physician discretion consistent with or different from best evidence;
- Patient preferences and compliance;
- Empirical evidence for variation;
- Insurance status prior to Medicare enrollment, dual eligibility, fee-for-service, Parts C and D Medicare; and
- Other factors deemed appropriate.

The effects of relevant sections of the Affordable Care and Budget Reconciliation Acts of 2010 on variation in Medicare Parts A, B, and C spending will be taken into account and recommendations made for changes in Medicare Parts A, B, and C payments for items and services that include impacts on physicians and hospitals, beneficiary access to care, and Medicare spending (but excluding graduate medical education, disproportionate share hospital, and health information technology add-ons).

The committee will further address whether Medicare payment systems should be modified to provide incentives for high-value, high-quality, evidence-based, patient-centered care through adoption of a value index (based on measures of quality and cost) that would adjust payments on a geographic area basis.

A workshop will be convened to gather public input into issues in the statement of task.

To meet a firm congressional deadline, a brief interim report will be issued in March 2013. The report will include the committee's preliminary observations, based primarily on the results of the sub-contracted analyses, but will not contain any recommendations.

A final report will be issued at the end of the project in approximately 36 months.

mensions (CMS, 2008; Conway, 2009; HHS, 2009; Porter, 2010; Wong et al., 2009). In legislation leading to this study, Congress defined high-value care as "the efficient delivery of high-quality, evidence-based, patient-centered care."[12] In traditional economic terms, "efficiency" is the production and allocation of goods and services that generate the greatest utility for a given set of resources or inputs, where "utility" reflects consumer satisfaction. As efficiency improves, more resources can be freed up to provide more goods and services.

In addition to deriving the greatest utility from a given set of inputs, economic efficiency reflects investing the proper amount of inputs into a given activity relative to other activities (Garber and Skinner, 2008). Thus, determining value in health care also requires having a measure of society's and/or an individual's willingness to pay for certain services relative to others. In the context of Medicare, this includes general coverage determinations, as well as specific reimbursement rates for covered items and services.

The goal of evaluating geographic variation in health care spending and quality imposed additional operational conditions on the definition of value. The measure of value would need to allow for comparisons of health care performance across different units of analysis using claims datasets. Consequently, the committee defined health care value as the equivalent of net benefit: *the amount by which overall health benefit and/or well-being produced by care exceeds (or falls short of) the costs of producing it.* Those costs should incorporate the opportunity costs of resources used to produce health care services. But because these opportunity costs seldom are observed directly, the committee defines "costs" for the purposes of this study as Medicare or other payer spending for goods and services. These observed costs are based on payment formulas that bear some relation to opportunity costs, but they could differ considerably.

To operationalize the committee's definition of value, consistency is necessary in the way health benefit is valued conceptually. Typically, either dollars or quality-adjusted life years (a measure of health outcomes) are used for this purpose. Because a health care system is designed to promote health through the provision of health care services, taking into account the system's fiscal sustainability,[13] health outcomes are a logical choice for assessing the overall health benefit or well-being attributable to health care. Health care researchers assess health outcomes using different quality metrics, which are intended to measure "the degree to which health [care] services for individuals and populations increase the likelihood of desired

---

[12]The Affordable Health Care for America Act, H.R. 3962, 111th Cong., 1st sess. (October 29, 2009).

[13]Expanding on an earlier definition of health care system purpose recommended by the Institute of Medicine (IOM, 2001).

health outcomes and are consistent with current professional knowledge" (IOM, 1990, p. 21). However, rarely is it straightforward to ascertain the contribution of an individual health care service to a specific health outcome, particularly in the management of chronic conditions. Measurement of health outcomes is challenging for numerous reasons, including those cited below and discussed in Chapter 2.

First, health is affected by determinants other than the provision of health care services, such as social factors, individual behavior, the environment, and genetics (McGinnis, 2002). Additionally, many health outcomes evolve over time and result from multiple patient-provider interactions across episodes of care. Consequently, attributing specific health outcomes to specific health care services or to individual providers can be difficult, especially in the context of chronic diseases or conditions.

Second, health is multidimensional. Thus, no single indicator accurately reflects a patient's overall health status. Although composite measures of health are available and in use, they are partial measures of health, as explained in Chapter 3. Moreover, "the perceived benefits of a particular intervention, diagnostic technology, or process will vary for each stakeholder in the health care system" (IOM, 2012a, p. 232).

Third, although a number of private organizations and government agencies have made tremendous progress toward developing health care quality metrics in recent decades, such metrics, especially those that purport to measure outcomes, still are not fully developed. Consequently, other metrics often are used to measure the performance of the health care system, and have been used successfully. For example, the Agency for Healthcare Research and Quality (AHRQ) endorses some process-of-care metrics that measure "health care-related activity performed for, on behalf of, or by a patient" if evidence indicates "that the clinical process ... has led to improved outcomes" (AHRQ, undated-a). Similar endorsements exist for specific structural and patient satisfaction metrics, where structure of care refers to "a feature of a health care organization or clinician related to the capacity to provide high quality health care," and patient satisfaction refers to "a patient's or enrollee's report of observations of and participation in health care, or assessment of any resulting change in their health" (AHRQ, undated-b).

The committee commends the efforts of public- and private-sector organizations such as AHRQ, the National Quality Forum, the National Committee for Quality Assurance, the Joint Commission, the American Medical Association, and CMS to advance the field of health care performance measurement and encourage public dissemination of results. As health outcome and cost measurement continues to improve in response to evolving technological capabilities and increasingly sophisticated, multidimensional metrics of health care performance, so, too, will the system's ability to encourage fiscal sustainability and high-quality care throughout the Medicare program and the U.S. health care system as a whole.

Statistical Analyses

Partly for reasons of data availability, the literature on geographic variation has focused on spending and utilization in traditional Medicare Parts A and B and, to a lesser extent, Part D. Little attention has been paid to the commercial health care sector, Medicare Advantage (also known as Part C), Medicaid, or the uninsured. To enhance current understanding of geographic variation, the committee commissioned empirical analyses of the complete database of Medicare beneficiaries, including Parts A, B, C, and D, as well as two nationwide commercial databases. These statistical analyses were focused on describing and accounting for geographic variation in health care spending, utilization, and quality; quantitative and qualitative syntheses of those analyses were performed as well. The committee additionally commissioned empirical analyses of Medicaid fee-for-service data, but the available samples were too small to enable reliable or valid statistical inferences, leading the committee to conclude that it would be inappropriate to draw any specific conclusions from the results. Consequently, the results of those analyses are not included in this report. Even more severe data limitations precluded meaningful analyses of geographic variation in spending among the uninsured, although the committee did attempt to account for this population in its analyses of total health care spending (see the related discussion in Chapter 2).

The following seven subcontractors supported the committee's core statistical analytic work: Acumen, LLC; Dartmouth Institute for Health Policy and Clinical Practice; Harvard University; The Lewin Group; Precision Health Economics, LLC; the RAND Corporation; and the University of Pittsburgh. Using large public and commercial claims databases (listed in Box 1-2), these subcontractors examined variation in aggregate health care spending, utilization, and quality across different units of analysis, including various geographic areas, as well as hospitals and providers. RAND modeled the impact of the committee's recommendations on providers, hospital referral regions, and total Medicare spending.

The subcontractors performed regression analyses to quantify how demographic, health status, and health plan characteristics of beneficiaries, as well as price and market factors, affect variation across geographic areas. In addition to the overall Medicare and commercial populations (aggregate analyses), 15 subpopulations with specific acute and chronic clinical conditions were studied (cohort analyses). The extent of geographic variation was examined within and across geographic units, across clinical condition cohorts, and over time. In accordance with CMS's direction, Medicare ex-

BOX 1-2
Commissioned Statistical Analyses

Subcontractor	Data Source
Acumen, LLC	Medicare Parts A, B, and D, as well as Medicare Advantage (Part C)*
Dartmouth Institute for Health Policy and Clinical Practice	Medicare Parts A and B (hospital-level data)
Harvard University	Thomson Reuters MarketScan Commercial Claims and Encounters database
The Lewin Group	Optum De-identified Normative Health Information (dNHI) database and Centers for Medicare & Medicaid Services (CMS) Chronic Conditions Warehouse database
Precision Health Economics, LLC	Synthesized data from the aforementioned analyses, as well as data on the uninsured
RAND Corporation	Medicare Parts A and B
University of Pittsburgh	Medicare Part D (prescription drug plans)

NOTE: For a complete description of these commissioned analyses, see Chapter 2.

*Analyses included all spending for dual-eligibles (by both Medicare and Medicaid) for Medicare-covered services.

SOURCE: All subcontractor spreadsheets and final reports can be accessed via the following link: http://www.iom.edu/geovariationmaterials.

penditures related to graduate medical education, disproportionate share hospitals, and indirect medical education were excluded from all spending calculations.

Additionally, because of issues of proprietary information and patient privacy, the committee was unable to access individual claims data used by the subcontractors. Consequently, the results presented in this report are based predominantly on aggregated output supplied by the subcontractors. The committee also contracted with two independent firms, IMPAQ International and RTI International, to perform a quality control audit of the research methods and statistical analyses applied to this study.

Public Workshops

The committee consulted with a number of experts and stakeholders through two public workshops and personal communications (see Appendix H for the workshop agendas). At the first public workshop, the committee heard testimony from the sponsor about the study scope. A member of Congress and congressional staff placed the study within its legislative context (Box 1-3 presents selected remarks made by these speakers). In addition, leading experts on geographic variation in health care spending and measurement of health care quality and value briefed the committee on the state of the science and evidence with regard to these topics.

At the second public workshop, the committee invited stakeholders to address the effects of geographic variation on their sectors or organizations. The 13 invited speakers represented the viewpoints of one or more of the following stakeholders: hospitals and health systems, clinicians, experts from organizations devoted to improving health care value, and consumers and purchasers. The discussion covered a range of topics relevant to the committee's scope of work, such as potential sources of geographic variation, methodological challenges entailed in measuring variation in spending and quality, and dimensions for consideration in determining payments. In addition, the committee heard testimony from members of the public. A formative discussion was held among many experts in the field, in which geographic variation was debated from numerous viewpoints. This discussion highlighted many topics that suggested domains of inquiry for this study.

Commissioned Papers

To complement its members' expertise, the committee commissioned papers from technical experts on the following topics:

- "Policy Approaches to Addressing Geographic Variation in Spending, Utilization, and High Value Care and the Implications of Those Approaches," by Marco D. Huesch, Michael K. Ong, and Dana P. Goldman
- "Economics Meets the Geography of Medicine," by Amitabh Chandra
- "Explaining Geographic Variation in Health Care Spending, Use and Quality, and Associated Methodological Challenges," by Willard G. Manning, Edward C. Norton, and Adam S. Wilk

---

BOX 1-3
Selected Testimony by Public Officials at the Committee's
Public Workshops (November 9, 2010)

Deputy Administrator of the Centers for Medicare
& Medicaid Services (CMS) Jonathan Blum

There are some who argue that much of the variation can't be explained. There are others who argue the variation can be explained when you take into account demographic considerations, teaching costs, disproportionate share costs. I think from our perspective, we are really hoping to build more consensus about what [are] the reasons and the causes and the impacts for health care spending variation, to help us develop policies to address those variations.

Member of the U.S. House of Representatives Allyson Schwartz

There were some in Congress who looked at geographic variation in spending, and believed that if we just smoothed out these differences by redistributing money from high cost areas to low cost areas, we could achieve greater value. I believe, in fact, it is not that simple. We all share the goal of promoting quality and reducing costs, but agreeing on what we mean by value and how best to achieve it prove to be pretty difficult.

Our goal is to ensure quality and improve health outcomes for the best price for all populations, and for good reasons. Spending may not be the same in every location or every population. Payment and delivery systems need not be the same. One size need not fit all. We do need to realign incentives for providers to drive cost efficiencies and quality improvement while maintaining incentives for teaching, innovation and medical advancement. We do need to learn from strategies that are working, including the many new delivery system innovations that will come from implementing health care reform. We need your help developing data that we can trust, data that appropriately reflects differing circumstances among providers, so that we can hold everyone account-

---

- "Geographic Variation in Health Care Spending and Utilization in Subgroups: Medicaid, Uninsured, and Undocumented Populations," by Ellen Meara

These papers contributed to the committee's deliberations and the evidentiary underpinnings of this report, although their perspectives and any implicit recommendations are solely those of the authors. These papers can be accessed on the IOM website at www.iom.edu/geovariationmaterials.

able to contain costs and to meet ongoing demands of a population that is aging, that is diverse, and that expects and deserves health care services that it needs.

Timothy Gronniger, Staff Member from the U.S.
House of Representatives' Subcommittee on Health
and Committee on Energy and Commerce

The value index at issue in this study, however, is clearly the geographic sort. With that in mind, the charge to your panel is to consider whether varying payments for defined geographic areas according to some measures of quality and cost is an appropriate next step for delivery system reform.

Geoff Gerhardt, Staff Member from the U.S. House of Representatives'
Subcommittee on Health and Committee on Ways and Means

Patient-based factors such as health status, ethnicity, income, education, treatment preferences, and presence of insurance may also help explain regional variation in spending patterns. Provider-based factors such as training, regional treatment norms, physician ownership, prevalence of fraud, and access to technology can play important roles in determining how much is spent in different areas. It is critical to recognize these types of factors when reaching conclusions about why spending and utilization vary from one part of the country to another.

Susan Walden, Staff Member from the U.S.
Senate's Committee on Finance

We should try to promote high value care, and the value payment modifier that [was] mentioned, that was enacted in the Senate bill which became law is an effort to do that for physicians primarily and in the fee-for-service system. But clearly the questions of how [to] measure quality and how [to] measure cost, those are the critical factors. Those are things that we look to the [Institute of Medicine] for your recommendations, because these are the most difficult.

Literature Search

In late 2010, the committee conducted an initial literature search of the following databases: MEDLINE, Embase, Scopus, Global Health, Web of Science, and Google Scholar, as well as several gray literature sources. Staff routinely updated the literature search and monitored electronic table of contents alerts from more than 20 journals throughout the course of this study. In all, the committee reviewed more than 2,500 peer-reviewed published articles. The committee relied on this literature to fill gaps in research areas that could not be addressed by the commissioned papers or subcontractors' empirical analyses.

REPORT STRUCTURE

This report comprises four chapters and is intended to be useful to both lay and technical audiences. Following this introduction and overview, Chapter 2 reports on the committee's commissioned statistical analyses and results, complemented by the findings of related literature on geographic variation in health care spending, utilization, and quality across the public and private health care sectors. Chapter 3 reviews proposals for adopting a geographically based value index for Medicare payments and presents the committee's statistical analytic findings that support rejection of the use of such an index. Finally, Chapter 4 considers various payment interventions for improving value throughout the U.S. health care system.

REFERENCES

AHRQ (Agency for Healthcare Research and Quality). undated-a. *National Quality Measures Clearinghouse: Domain framework and inclusion criteria.* http://www.qualitymeasures. ahrq.gov/about/domain-definitions.aspx (accessed July 12, 2013).

————. undated-b. *National Quality Measures Clearinghouse: Varieties of measures in NQMC.* http://www.qualitymeasures.ahrq.gov/tutorial/varieties.aspx (accessed July 12, 2013).

Baicker, K., and A. Chandra. 2004. Medicare spending, the physician workforce, and beneficiaries' quality of care. *Health Affairs* Supplemental Web Exclusives W4-184-97.

CBO (Congressional Budget Office). 2008. *Key issues in analyzing major health insurance proposals.* Washington, DC: CBO.

CMS (Centers for Medicare & Medicaid Services). 2008. *Roadmap for implementing value driven healthcare in the traditional medicare fee-for-service program.* Baltimore, MD: CMS.

————. 2013. *National health expenditure data: Historical.* http://www.cms.gov/Research-Statistics-Data-and-Systems/Statistics-Trends-and-Reports/NationalHealthExpendData/NationalHealthAccountsHistorical.html (accessed May 7, 2013).

Conway, P. H. 2009. Value-driven health care: Implications for hospitals and hospitalists. *Journal of Hospital Medicine* 4(8):507-511.

Dartmouth Institute for Health Policy and Clinical Practice. 2013. *The Dartmouth Atlas of Health Care.* http://www.dartmouthatlas.org (accessed July 18, 2013).

Docteur, E., and R. A. Berenson. 2009. *How does the quality of U.S. health care compare internationally? Timely analysis of immediate health policy issues.* Washington, DC: The Urban Institute.

Fisher, E. S., D. E. Wennberg, T. A. Stukel, D. J. Gottlieb, F. L. Lucas, and E. L. Pinder. 2003a. The implications of regional variations in Medicare spending. Part 1: The content, quality, and accessibility of care. *Annals of Internal Medicine* 138(4):273-287.

————. 2003b. The implications of regional variations in Medicare spending. Part 2: Health outcomes and satisfaction with care. *Annals of Internal Medicine* 138(4):288-298.

Garber, A. M., and J. Skinner. 2008. Is American health care uniquely inefficient? *Journal of Economic Perspectives* 22(4):27-50.

HHS (U.S. Department of Health and Human Services). 2009. *Value-driven health care home.* http://www.hhs.gov/valuedriven (accessed July 18, 2013).

IOM (Institute of Medicine). 1990. *Medicare: A strategy for quality assurance, Volume II.* Washington, DC: National Academy Press.

———. 1999. *To err is human: Building a safer health system.* Edited by J. M. Corrigan, M. S. Donaldson and L. T. Kohn. Washington, DC: National Academy Press.

———. 2001. *Crossing the quality chasm: A new health system for the 21st century.* Washington, DC: National Academy Press.

———. 2002. *Leadership by example: Coordinating government roles in improving health care quality.* Washington, DC: The National Academies Press.

———. 2003. *Priority areas for national action: Transforming health care quality.* Washington, DC: The National Academies Press.

———. 2006a. *Performance measurement: Accelerating improvement.* Washington, DC: The National Academies Press.

———. 2006b. *Rewarding provider performance: Aligning incentives in Medicare.* Washington, DC: The National Academies Press.

———. 2010a. *The healthcare imperative: Lowering costs and improving outcomes.* Washington, DC: The National Academies Press.

———. 2010b. *Value in health care: Accounting for cost, quality, safety, outcomes, and innovation: Workshop summary.* Edited by P. L. Young, L. Olsen, and J. M. McGinnis. Washington, DC: The National Academies Press.

———. 2011. *Geographic adjustment in Medicare payment—Phase I: Improving accuracy.* Washington, DC: The National Academies Press.

____. 2012a. *Best care at lower cost: The path to continuously learning health care in America.* Washington, DC: The National Academies Press.

———. 2012b. *Geographic adjustment in Medicare payment—Phase II: Implications for access, quality, and efficiency.* Washington, DC: The National Academies Press.

Kaiser Family Foundation. 2012. *Health care costs: A primer. Key information on health care costs and their impact.* Washington, DC: Kaiser Family Foundation.

Levinson, D. R. 2010. *Adverse events in hospitals: National incidence among Medicare beneficiaries.* Washington, DC: Department of Health and Human Services, Office of the Inspector General.

McGinnis, J. M., P. Williams-Russo, and J. R. Knickman. 2002. The case for more active policy attention to health promotion. *Health Affairs* 21(2):78-92.

MedPAC (Medicare Payment Advisory Commission). 2007. Promoting greater efficiency in Medicare. In *Report to the Congress: June 2007.* Washington, DC: MedPAC.

———. 2009. Measuring regional variation in service use. In *Report to the Congress: December 2009.* Washington, DC: MedPAC.

———. 2011. Regional variation in Medicare service use. In *Report to the Congress: January 2011.* Washington, DC: MedPAC.

ModernHealthcare.com. 2013. *CBO projects less growth in healthcare spending.* http://www.modernhealthcare.com/article/20130515/NEWS/305159959?AllowView=VW8xUmo5Q21TcWJOb1gzb0tNN3RLZ0h0MWg5SVgra3NZRzROR3l0WWRMWGJVZndFRWxiNUtpQzMyWmV1NW5rWUpibW8=&utm_source=link-20130515-NEWS-305159959&utm_medium=email&utm_campaign=mpdaily (accessed May 15, 2013).

National Governors Association and National Association of State Budget Officers. 2012. *The fiscal survey of states.* Washington, DC: National Governors Association and the National Association of State Budget Officers.

NRC (National Research Council). 2010. *Accounting for health and health care: Approaches to measuring the sources and costs of their improvement.* Washington, DC: The National Academies Press.

Porter, M. E. 2010. What is value in health care? *New England Journal of Medicine* 363(26): 2477-2481.

Schoen, C., A. K. Fryer, S. R. Collins, and D. C. Radley. 2011. *State trends in premiums and deductibles, 2003-2010: The need for action to address rising costs.* Washington, DC: The Commonwealth Fund.

Sebelius, K. 2010. Letter to the Quality Care Coalition, March 20, 2010. Washington, DC: The Secretary of Health and Human Services.

Skinner, J., D. Staiger, and E. S. Fisher. 2010. Looking back, moving forward. *New England Journal of Medicine* 362(7):569-574.

Social Security and Medicare Boards of Trustees. 2008. *Status of the Social Security and Medicare programs.* Washington, DC: Social Security and Medicare Boards of Trustees.

The Pew Center on the States. 2012. *The widening gap.* Washington, DC: The Pew Institute.

Wennberg, J. E., and M. M. Cooper. 1999. *The quality of medical care in the United States: A report on the Medicare program. The Dartmouth Atlas of Health Care 1999.* Hanover, NH, and Chicago, IL: Darmouth Medical School and American Hospital Association.

Wennberg, J. E., E. S. Fisher, and J. S. Skinner. 2002. Geography and the debate over Medicare reform. *Health Affairs* Supplemental Web Exclusives W96-W114.

Wong, J. B., C. Mulrow, and H. C. Sox. 2009. Health policy and cost-effectiveness analysis: Yes we can. Yes we must. *Annals of Internal Medicine* 150(4):274-275.

World Bank. 2012. *Data: Health expenditure per capita (current US$).* http://data.worldbank.org/indicator/SH.XPD.PCAP (accessed December 2012).

Zhang, Y., K. Baicker, and J. P. Newhouse. 2010. Geographic variation in the quality of prescribing. *New England Journal of Medicine* 363(21):1985-1988.

2

Empirical Analysis of Geographic Variation

As described in Chapter 1, the Centers for Medicare & Medicaid Services (CMS) charged the Institute of Medicine's (IOM's) Committee on Geographic Variation in Health Care Spending and Promotion of High-Value Care with examining "geographic variation in intensity, cost, and growth of health care services and in per capita health care spending among the Medicare, Medicaid, privately insured, and uninsured U.S. populations." To this end, the committee commissioned new analyses to complement its evaluation of the existing literature. The purpose of these new analyses was to quantify the magnitude of geographic variation in spending, utilization, and quality across various populations, payers, and geographic units; to evaluate known (and measurable) factors that account for variation in the Medicare and commercial markets; and to identify types of health care services with disproportionately high rates of variation that drive total variation.

RESEARCH FRAMEWORK AND STATISTICAL MODELING APPROACH

The literature on geographic variation has focused largely on traditional, fee-for-service Medicare. Much less is known about variation in expenditures and outcomes in the private market and in other public programs, such as Medicaid and Medicare Advantage (also known as Medicare Part C). This gap in knowledge is significant. A recent study notes that in 2010, Medicare spending accounted for 23 percent of the $2.19 trillion spent on personal health care in the United States, while spending in the private sector and Medicaid made up 34 and 17 percent, respectively (MedPAC, 2012). Although Medicare beneficiaries represent just 15 percent of the total U.S. population, more than 60 percent of Americans are covered by private insurance (ASPE, 2011). Moreover, 28 percent of all Medicare beneficiaries are enrolled in the Medicare Advantage program, which allows private insurers to contract with CMS to provide Medicare-covered Part A, B, and D services (Gold et al., 2013). Medicare is the largest single payer for health care in the nation, and has for many years been the only available source of reliable national claims data (Bernstein et al., 2011; Reschovsky et al., 2011). Nonetheless, spending and utilization patterns in traditional Medicare should not be assumed to be representative of other payer markets or of total U.S. health care spending and utilization.

To better understand the causes of variation in the health care system, the committee commissioned original empirical analyses of the complete database of Medicare beneficiaries (by Acumen, LLC; Dartmouth Institute of Health Policy and Clinical Practice; and the University of Pittsburgh), as well as two nationwide commercial databases, OptumInsight (by The Lewin Group) and Thomson Reuters (TR) MarketScan (by Harvard University).[1,2] The results of these analyses were synthesized and used to conduct a separate analysis of geographic variation in total health care spending (by Precision Health Economics, LLC [PHE]).

The subcontractors conducted a series of regression and correlation analyses to examine geographic variation in spending, utilization, and quality among the overall Medicare and commercial populations (aggregate analyses), as well as among 15 subpopulations with acute and chronic clinical conditions (cohort analyses). As noted in Chapter 1, not all geographic variation is unacceptable. The analyses conducted for this study generally excluded acceptable variation, which occurs as a result of factors beyond the control of the health care system in a region. Specifically, the baseline regression model was used to examine geographic variation in spending and utilization, adjusted for input prices of areas, as well as the age, sex, and health status of patients. As detailed in later sections, except where noted, regression models were not adjusted for other factors beyond the

---

[1]Two different commercial databases were used to improve the external validity of the analyses of variation in the private sector. Each database had unique advantages: While the TR MarketScan database is large and representative, the OptumInsight database provides rich, individual-level data on a number of demographic factors. Results for both commercial populations are presented throughout Chapter 2 and 3, alongside the Medicare findings. For details on each database, refer to Appendix C and the subcontractor reports. (All subcontractor final reports and spreadsheets of results are publicly available on the IOM webpage at http://www.iom.edu/geovariationmaterials.)

[2]Refer to Chapter 1, Box 1-2, for a complete list of subcontractors performing these analyses and corresponding data sources.

control of the health care system that often are associated with poor health status or higher spending, such as beneficiaries' race and income, or factors that cannot be measured using claims data, such as patient or physician preferences. The specific research methodologies of these analyses are summarized in Appendix C and further detailed in the individual subcontractor reports. The results of the empirical analyses are presented in this chapter and Chapter 3.

The committee also commissioned analyses of the Medicaid database (by Acumen, LLC). As noted in Chapter 1, however, those findings are not presented in this report because of concerns about their reliability and validity due to incomplete data. The Acumen report notes that in 2007, more than 64 percent of all Medicaid beneficiaries were at least partially covered by a managed care program. Data on these beneficiaries had large gaps, as CMS did not begin collecting encounter claims data on managed care enrollees until 2012 (Acumen, LLC, 2013a). In addition, studies of Medicaid generally are restricted to populations enrolled in fee-for-service programs, thus limiting the reliability and generalizability of results based on Medicaid data (Autor et al., 2011). Unlike Medicare, moreover, Medicaid can vary considerably in programming and policies because states can request waivers from CMS to operate outside of federal guidelines. Medicaid programming and policies also have changed over time, so the data available for individual states vary widely. As described below, however, PHE imputed values for a hospital referral region's (HRR's) Medicaid population in its calculation of total U.S. health care spending.

The committee's analysis of geographic variation for the uninsured population also was restricted. According to the 2011 Current Population Survey, the uninsured population, one in seven of whom is an undocumented immigrant, made up approximately 16 percent of the total U.S. population in 2010 (ASPE, 2011; Zuckerman et al., 2011). Although uninsurance rates are known to vary greatly among states, a comprehensive analysis of geographic variation among the uninsured could not be conducted because of the lack of a coordinated database on the financing and delivery of care for this population. As discussed in later sections of this chapter, however, PHE adjusted its calculation of total U.S. health care spending, and associated analyses of variation for spending incurred by the uninsured were conducted using census data and Medical Expenditure Panel Survey (MEPS) data (PHE, 2013).

This chapter presents findings from the committee's empirical evaluation of geographic variation, with support from the existing literature. After briefly addressing the methodological issue of the unit of analysis, the chapter confirms the robust presence of regional variation in both Medicare and commercial health care spending and utilization across multiple geographic units as well as over time. It then explores the sources of this geographic variation, evaluating the role of price; other patient-, provider-, and market-level factors also are examined. Next, the influence of high variation in post-acute care services on total variation in Medicare spending and utilization is discussed. Finally, the chapter briefly assesses the limitations of efforts to analyze variation in quality and presents the committee's recommendation for future research.

GEOGRAPHIC VARIATION AND THE UNIT OF ANALYSIS

The performance of the health care system varies across different units of analysis, including physician, practice, health care system, and geographic unit. Geographic units can in turn be defined by economic markets (e.g., HRRs), political boundaries (e.g., county, state), administrative areas (e.g., zip codes, census tracts), or where people live (e.g., metropolitan statistical areas). In accordance with its statement of task, the committee examined variation within "areas of different sizes" to determine how variation is affected by different levels of aggregation. Box 2-1 defines technical geographic units referenced throughout the literature on geographic variation and this report. To the extent possible, the committee considered variation across and within individual providers in an area, although in practice, concerns about patient privacy, proprietary information, and small sample sizes precluded public release of analyses at the individual physician level (and even results pertaining to small geographic areas).

CONFIRMING REGIONAL VARIATION IN
SPENDING AND UTILIZATION

Health care spending is a measure of expenditures for care, and reflects the effects of both the utilization of health services and their prices. "Utilization" captures the total number of units or intensity of health care services, as well as the mix of services provided. Recent reports by the Dartmouth Institute for Health Policy and Clinical Practice and the Medicare Payment Advisory Commission (MedPAC) estimate that unadjusted Medicare spending per beneficiary is 50-55 percent higher in HRRs in the highest quintile of spending relative to those in the lowest quintile. Medicare service use (adjusted for demographics and beneficiary health) is approximately 30 percent greater in the highest quintile compared with the lowest (MedPAC, 2011; Zuckerman et al., 2010). These findings are corroborated by a large body of literature that highlights the robust presence of variation in health care spending and utilization across regions in the United States (CBO, 2008; Fisher and Wennberg, 2003; Fisher et al., 2003a,b; GAO, 2009; MedPAC, 2003, 2009; Wennberg et al., 2002, 2008).

BOX 2-1
Definitions of Geographic Units Frequently Used
in Health Services Research

- *Hospital service areas (HSAs)*—Created by Dartmouth and defined by assigning to an HSA the zip codes from which a hospital or several hospitals draw the greatest proportion of their Medicare patients. There are 3,426 HSAs (Dartmouth Institute for Health Policy and Clinical Practice, 2013).

- *Hospital referral regions (HRRs)*—Created by Dartmouth to represent regional health care markets for tertiary (complex) medical care. Dartmouth defined 306 HRRs by assigning HSAs to regions where the greatest proportion of major cardiovascular procedures were performed, "with minor modifications to achieve geographic contiguity, a minimum total population size of 120,000, and a high localization index" (Dartmouth Institute for Health Policy and Clinical Practice, 2013).

- *Metropolitan statistical areas (MSAs, or metropolitan core-based statistical areas [CBSAs])*—Created by the Office of Management and Budget using counties. Each of 388 MSAs (OMB, 2013) includes one or more counties with one core urban area of 50,000 individuals or more, as well as "adjacent counties exhibiting a high degree of social and economic integration" (as measured by such factors as commuting patterns) with an urban core (OMB, 2010). Areas that do not qualify as MSAs are often classified as "outside" MSAs (OMB, 2010) or non-MSAs. The Centers for Medicare & Medicaid Services (CMS) adjusts hospital payments according to a hospital wage index calculated for MSAs and non-MSAs* (CMS, 2012).

---

*CBSAs are geographic entities that the Office of Management and Budget implemented in 2003 (OMB, 2010). The committee's commissioned analyses used MSAs (a subcomponent of CBSAs also referred to as metropolitan CBSAs), as well as non-MSA "rest of state" regions. For simplicity, and in accordance with expert practice in this area (Acumen, LLC, 2009; MedPAC, 2012; OMB, 2010), the committee uses the term "metropolitan CBSA" throughout this report.

Medicare and Commercial Spending Varies
Across All Levels of Geography

For the present study, variation was examined at three geographic units of measurement: hospital service area (HSA), HRR, and metropolitan core-based statistical area (metropolitan CBSA). In the Acumen Medicare analysis, total spending, measured per capita, includes all costs incurred (by beneficiary and insurer) in traditional fee-for-service Medicare (Parts A, B, and D). Medicare Advantage (Part C) was evaluated in a separate analysis discussed below. Similarly, in the OptumInsight (Lewin) and MarketScan (Harvard) analyses of commercial data, total spending includes all facility, provider, and prescription drug costs incurred by the beneficiary, the insurer, and any additional (secondary) payers. To keep the presentation manageable, the analysis results are shown as a summary measure of variation—the 90th percentile of spending compared with the 10th percentile (for aggregated years 2007-2009). This value is approximately the ratio of average spending in the highest-spending quintile of geographic units to average spending in the lowest-spending quintile.

The analysis results, displayed in Table 2-1, show that without adjustments for any differences among regions, the HRR in the 90th percentile spent 42 percent more per Medicare beneficiary each month than the HRR in the 10th percentile. At the metropolitan CBSA level, the 90th percentile spent 38 percent more than the 10th percentile per beneficiary each month. Similar analyses of commercial insurance data confirm the presence of spending variation for all geographic units.

Table 2-1 also shows that considerably greater variation exists at the smaller, HSA level. The policy implications of increasing levels of variation for smaller geographic units are discussed in Chapter 4. The committee, however, has chosen to present analysis results at the HRR level in the remainder of this report, as the corresponding area served by a major tertiary care hospital is the most widely established unit of analysis in the literature on geographic variation.

TABLE 2-1
Ratio of the 90th to the 10th Percentiles of Unadjusted[a] Per-Member-Per Month (PMPM) Medicare and Commercial Spending Across Geographic Units

	HSA	HRR	Metropolitan CBSA
Medicare	1.47	1.42	1.38
Commercial 1 (OptumInsight)	1.71[b]	1.42	1.50
Commercial 2 (MarketScan)	1.43	1.36	1.36

NOTE: Metropolitan CBSA = metropolitan core-based statistical area (also referred to as metropolitan statistical area [MSA]); HRR = hospital referral region; HSA = hospital service area.

[a]"Unadjusted spending" refers to all-cause spending that has not been adjusted for any factors other than year of analysis and length of beneficiary enrollment.

[b]The OptumInsight results in this table are based on 2,896 HSAs with at least 500 observations. The analysis was conducted using only "large" HSAs to mitigate the effect of outliers. The Medicare and MarketScan databases were much larger; the data generally had normal distribution and were less affected by outliers.

SOURCE: Committee analysis of subcontractor data.

While variation occurs for all levels of geography, public- and private-sector spending per beneficiary (adjusted for age, sex, and health status) are only weakly correlated at the HRR level (PHE, 2013). In other words, areas that are high spenders in Medicare are not necessarily high spenders in the commercial market and vice versa. As shown in Table 2-2, the two commercial databases correlate well with each other, but are weakly correlated with Medicare. As described in later sections, spending variation in Medicare is driven by variation in utilization of post-acute services, whereas in the commercial population, price has a greater influence than utilization on overall spending variation.

As noted previously, most of the literature on geographic variation has of necessity relied on data from Medicare Parts A and B. Any measure of total spending by HRR is necessarily incomplete because of data limitations but is useful as a measure of the total resources potentially available to medical decision makers in an HRR. It is surprising that the correlation of Medicare spending with total spending is not higher (see Table 2-3), as Medicare accounts for a substantial fraction of total health care spending. Moreover, it is unclear why a phenomenon responsible for variation

TABLE 2-2
Correlation of Spending Measures Between Medicare and Commercial Payers

	Medicare & MarketScan	Medicare & OptumInsight	MarketScan & OptumInsight
"Raw"[a] Baseline Spending	0.112	0.081	0.663
Input Price Adjusted Baseline Spending	-0.094	-0.032	0.632

NOTE: All hospital referral region means are from the "Baseline" regression model, and thereby adjusted for partial year enrollment, age, sex, age*sex, and health status.

[a]"Raw" spending refers to all-cause spending not adjusted for input-prices.

SOURCE: PHE, 2013.

TABLE 2-3
Correlation Between Total Spending and Payer-Specific Spending

	MarketScan	Medicare
Total Spending (Input Price Adjusted)	0.21	0.30

SOURCE: PHE, 2013.

in Medicare expenditures, such as practice patterns, would not matter for total spending as well. A map showing PHE's estimate of quintiles of total spending across HRRs is included in Appendix G.

The committee commissioned a separate analysis of variation in Medicare Advantage (Part C) spending. That analysis was limited in scope as individual-level claims data were not available for the 2007-2009 study period; therefore, the analysis examined spending variation based on total monthly Medicare reimbursement paid to Medicare Advantage plans (Acumen, LLC, 2013a).[3] In part because of a policy decision to raise reimbursements in HRRs with lower traditional Medicare spending, the analysis found somewhat less variation in Medicare Advantage spending compared with traditional Medicare: HRRs in the 90th percentile spent 36 percent more per Medicare Advantage beneficiary than HRRs in the 10th percentile, while Table 2-1 shows a slightly higher differential ratio for fee-for-service beneficiaries. The distribution of the 90th to the 10th HRR cost percentile is narrower, as Medicare Advantage monthly spending is based on benchmarks set by the Congress. Although average per capita spending is higher for Medicare Advantage ($986) than for traditional Medicare ($958), HRR-level expenditures are correlated between the two programs (0.66).

A complementary analysis by PHE examined geographic variation in total health care spending at the HRR level. This measure accounts for the total population in the United States by synthesizing estimates from Acumen's population-specific study of Medicare and Medicaid fee-for-service (Acumen, LLC, 2013a,b) and Harvard's analysis of the MarketScan database as a proxy for commercial spending (Harvard University, 2012). Spending for the uninsured population was imputed by estimating a factor price-adjusted national average based on census and MEPS data. The spending estimate for Medicaid Managed Care was generated using enrollment and total dollars paid for Medicaid health maintenance organization (HMO) beneficiaries by state, using data from the Medicaid Statistical Information System (MSIS). To create the total spending measure, payer-specific weights were applied.[4] The analysis of total spending found that HRRs in the 90th percentile spend 50 percent more per beneficiary each month than HRRs in the 10th percentile, a larger variation than that shown in Table 2-1 for Medicare or commercial insurers (PHE, 2013).

---

[3]CMS began collecting individual encounter claims data for Medicare Advantage beneficiaries in April 2012.

[4]See PHE (2013) for detailed methodology. That report is publicly available on the IOM webpage at the following link: http://www.iom.edu/geovariationmaterials.

Medicare and Commercial Utilization of Health Care Varies Across Service Categories

The committee also commissioned analyses of geographic variation in utilization, which is measured in two ways. The first entails measuring utilization as "counts" of specific medical services, such as the number of emergency department and office visits per beneficiary per month. Because there are many different types of services, any measure of total utilization must be a weighted sum of those services (for example, a hospital day should count more than a single laboratory test). The subcontractors weighted each service by a standard national price for that service to remove the effect of different prices across geographic locations and derive a measure of the aggregate quantity of services. This is the second measure of total utilization.[5]

The ratios of the 90th to the 10th percentile of risk-adjusted utilization (measured as counts) point to the presence of regional variation across different types of health care services within both the Medicare and commercial payer populations (see Table 2-4). The high use of emergency department services among the MarketScan commercial population is particularly striking, as utilization among HRRs in the 90th percentile (measured as counts of visits per beneficiary per month) is more than twice as high as that among HRRs in the 10th percentile.

A recent MedPAC analysis also reveals substantial regional variation in service-specific utilization. Metropolitan CBSAs in the 90th percentile utilized approximately 2.01 times as much post-acute care per beneficiary as metropolitan CBSAs in the 10th percentile (MedPAC, 2011).[6] After post-acute care services, the ambulatory care (outpatient visit) and inpatient visit categories varied the most, with 90th to 10th percentile ratios of 1.24 and 1.22, respectively (MedPAC, 2011). The impact of post-acute care services on variation in total Medicare spending and utilization is discussed in greater detail later in this chapter.

The wide variation in inpatient hospitalization spending has been a key focus in the literature. Findings have shown that these regional differences may result from variation in the per capita rates of admission and readmission (Fisher et al., 1994; Wennberg and Cooper, 1998), average lengths of hospital stay (Yuan et al., 2000), and mix of patient diagnosis-related groups (DRGs) (Frick et al., 1985; Steinwald, 2003), and indirectly from

---

[5]Refer to Appendix E for detail on the methodology.

[6]This MedPAC analysis adjusts for input price and health status. The MedPAC report notes that this regression model used a "service sector-specific health status adjustor. For example, metastatic cancer would have a much greater coefficient for total service utilization than it would for post acute care. This is different than using a beneficiary's HCC [hierarchical condition category] score to adjust for health status" (MedPAC, 2011, p. 7).

TABLE 2-4
Ratio of the 90th to the 10th Percentile of Per-Member-Per Month (PMPM)
Risk-Adjusted Utilization (measured as counts) of Selected[a] Service Categories
Among Medicare and Commercial Populations at the Hospital Referral Region Level

	Inpatient Admission	Outpatient Visits	Prescription Drug Fills	Emergency Department Visits	Imaging Procedures
Medicare	1.29	1.33	1.19	1.33	1.23
Commercial 1 (OptumInsight)	1.48	1.46	1.36	1.54	1.76
Commercial 2 (MarketScan)	1.45	1.30	1.34	2.04	1.33

NOTE: Utilization figures have been adjusted for age, sex, and health status.

[a]The committee was limited in the number of utilization measures it could investigate across Medicare and commercial databases due to time and budget constraints. Hence, post-acute care was not included in the committee's main analysis. However, upon receiving preliminary results of the analysis, the committee asked Acumen to investigate post-acute care. Commercial payers did not conduct a similar analysis due to their younger populations, who receive very little post-acute care as a population. This table only presents utilization measures that are common across payer populations.

SOURCE: Committee analysis of subcontractor data.

a host of inpatient-care and efficiency-related factors (nurse staffing, tests, procedures, drugs) that may differ across and within geographic regions (Franzini et al., 2010).

The empirical analyses of Medicare and commercial data demonstrate considerable variation in emergency department and outpatient visits. This variation may be due to underlying differences in the regional distribution of socioeconomic factors shown to influence emergency department use (Cunningham, 2006). Significant regional variation also may exist in the organizational structure of emergency response staff, as well as the technical capacity of emergency department facilities (Cummins, 1993) and/or the supply and availability of primary care services (Cunningham, 2006).

The University of Pittsburgh analysis of Medicare Part D found HRR-level variation in prescription drug spending and use,[7] with 90th to 10th percentile ratios of 1.24 and 1.17, respectively (University of Pittsburgh, 2013). Although a multitude of studies have assessed variation in total utilization of health care, the literature on variation in the use of prescription drugs is limited.

---

[7]The Pittsburgh analysis adjusted drug spending for patient demographics (age, sex, race, income), insurance status, and clinical characteristics (CMS-HCC risk scores, prescription drug HCC [RxHCC] risk scores, and institutionalization status) (University of Pittsburgh, 2013, p. 9).

Geographic Variation Persists Over Time

Although total health care spending has grown steadily over time (Fisher et al., 2009), Figure 2-1 demonstrates that in the past four decades, per capita health care spending has been growing more rapidly in the commercial sector than in Medicare. The committee commissioned "growth" analyses to assess whether geographic variation persists over time, and thus can be considered a true signal rather than a result of random noise. At any fixed point in time, area-level expenditures reflect the underlying spending habits of individual beneficiaries while also reflecting some degree of random noise arising from the uncertainty of individual health episodes. The former factor persists over time, while the latter does not. Trends in prices paid by commercial insurers and the demographics of those whom they insure also may change over time in ways that do not mimic Medicare.

Acumen's analysis of Medicare data found that spending and utilization growth rates have not differed much over time between high- and low-cost regions of the country; regions that were high- (or low-) cost in 1992 remained so in 2010 (Acumen, LLC, 2013b). This finding is illustrated in Figure 2-2, which classifies HRRs into cost quintiles based on their expenditure levels in 1992; quintiles 1 and 5 represent the lowest- and highest-cost regions, respectively. After regional differences due to input price, age, sex, and health status are removed, expenditure growth patterns are highly similar in each quintile (with the exception of some regression toward the mean for quintile 5). In short, spending differences between low- and high-cost geographic regions persist over time and thus do not simply reflect random variation at a point in time. Utilization growth rates mirror the spending patterns presented in Figure 2-2. These results are consistent with the existing literature, which reports that variation in Medicare spending persists across areas over time (Cutler and Sheiner, 1999).

Another demonstration of the stability of the HRR cost quintiles over time is shown in Tables 2-5 and 2-6, which display the change in quintile rank between 1992 and 2010 for spending and utilization, respectively (Acumen, LLC, 2013b). As shown in Table 2-5, among all HRRs in the lowest-cost quintile of spending in 1992, 61 percent remained in the lowest-cost quintile in 2010, 28 percent moved to the second-lowest-cost quintile, and so on. Stability in utilization, displayed in Table 2-6, is weaker, with only 46 percent of HRRs in the lowest-cost quintile remaining in that quintile in 2010.

As a final way of distinguishing the portion of geographic variation that arises from systematic differences and the portion that is random, the subcontractors examined correlations of year-to-year spending and year-to-year utilization during 1992 and 2010 (Acumen, LLC, 2013b). Area-level Medicare spending is highly correlated from one year to the next, with an

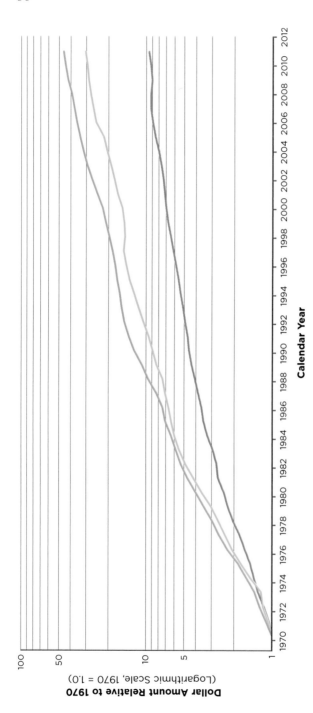

Calendar Year

GDP Per Capita
Medicare $ Per Enrollee
Private Health Insurance $ Per Enrollee

FIGURE 2-1 Cumulative growth in spending for Medicare and private health insurance per enrollee compared with growth in per capita gross domestic product (GDP) between 1970 and 2012.

SOURCE: Committee analysis of national health expenditure data.

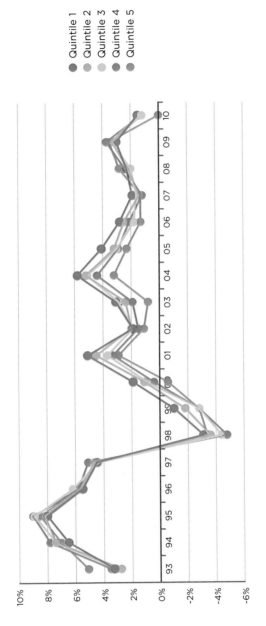

FIGURE 2-2 Growth rates of Medicare spending, adjusted for demographics, health status, and input price, among quintiles[a] of hospital referral regions (HRRs) based on expenditure levels in 1992.

[a]The same HRRs are included in each cost quintile throughout the period of analysis. Quintiles 1 and 5 represent the lowest and highest cost regions, respectively.

SOURCE: Acumen, LLC, 2013b.

TABLE 2-5
Stability in Medicare Spending Quintiles

Quintile in 1992	Quintile in 2010				
	1	2	3	4	5
1 (lowest)	61%	28%	10%	2%	0%
2	26%	41%	23%	7%	3%
3	13%	21%	38%	25%	3%
4	0%	8%	23%	44%	25%
5 (highest)	0%	2%	7%	23%	69%

SOURCE: Acumen, LLC, 2013b.

TABLE 2-6
Stability in Medicare Utilization Quintiles

Quintile in 1992	Quintile in 2010				
	1	2	3	4	5
1 (lowest)	46%	25%	16%	8%	5%
2	30%	33%	23%	13%	2%
3	21%	25%	25%	16%	13%
4	2%	13%	30%	33%	23%
5 (highest)	2%	5%	7%	29%	58%

SOURCE: Acumen, LLC, 2013b.

average Pearson correlation of 0.96 between any given year "t" and year "t + 5" (for example, between 1992 and 1997). Year-to-year Medicare utilization is slightly less correlated, with a Pearson correlation of 0.86 for any given year "t" and year "t + 5." These high correlations are further evidence that HRR spending and utilization levels are stable, with regions that are high- (or low-) cost in 1992 remaining so in 2010. In other words, little of the variation is random. More precisely, random variation in average HRR-level Medicare spending in any one year is small relative to the mean (ranging from 2 percent for the largest HRR to 4 percent for the smallest HRR), suggesting that sample sizes per HRR are sufficiently large to support conclusions.

Acumen's Medicare Advantage analysis also found a strong correlation of spending over time (2007-2009 period of analysis), with correlation coefficients greater than 0.972 for all year-to-year comparisons (Acumen, LLC, 2013a). As noted earlier, Medicare Advantage spending is highly stable as it is determined by CMS benchmarks, which are based on historical fee-for-service rates and updated yearly. The Harvard MarketScan analysis echoes the Medicare growth analysis, finding moderately high correlations (ranging from 0.68 to 0.88) of area-level year-to-year commercial spending during 2006 and 2010 (Harvard University, 2012). Naturally, correlations drop as intervals between years increase; for example, the correlation of spending between 2006 and 2007 is 0.77, whereas that between 2006 and 2010 is 0.57. Overall, the high year-to-year correlation and quintile stability suggest that geographic variation is real and not an artifact of random noise.

Conclusion 2.1. Geographic variation in spending and utilization is real, and not an artifact reflecting random noise. The committee's empirical analyses of Medicare and commercial data confirm the robust presence of variation, which persists across geographic units and health care services and over time.

THE ROLE OF VARIATION IN PRICE

As discussed earlier, variation in health care spending reflects variation in both price and utilization (quantity of services). Price is the amount paid by insurers and beneficiaries to a provider per unit of health care services. Price variation is attributable to two factors: (1) differences in the prices of inputs that are beyond a provider's control (costs related to capital; labor; and other overhead costs, such as rent and insurance), and (2) the margin above the cost of inputs that a payer or provider chooses to set or negotiate (Gold, 2004). Whereas CMS traditionally sets a uniform national base price, adjusting for the differences in input prices across geographic areas and certain other factors, commercial prices are set through negotiations between payers and providers (Chernew et al., 2010; Dunn et al., 2012). Because negotiating power varies across areas, the variation in prices received by providers is substantially larger in the commercial sector than in Medicare.

Analyses conducted for this study support the results in the existing literature, which reports that adjusting for regional differences in prices has little effect on observed variation in Medicare spending (Cutler and Sheiner, 1999; Fuchs et al., 2001; Gottlieb et al., 2010). In this study, adjustments for input prices slightly increased geographic variation as compared with unadjusted spending. HRR-level input-price-adjusted spending at the 90th percentile was 44 percent more per Medicare beneficiary than input-price-adjusted spending at the 10th percentile.[8] However, this does not imply that the HRRs in the 90th and 10th percentiles of unadjusted spending and input-price-adjusted spending are the same. In other words, a high-spending HRR could hypothetically move to a low-spending quintile following the elimination of regional variation due to input prices.

In the commercial market, however, regional differences in price rather than utilization of health care services influence much of the overall regional variation in spending (Donohue et al., 2012; Dunn et al., 2012). In the MarketScan commercial population, adjustment for input prices reduced variation across areas by only a small amount, as the difference between the 90th and 10th percentiles of spending decreased from 36 percent to 33 percent (Harvard University, 2012). To further explore the effects of price, Harvard's MarketScan analysis examined relationships among spending, quantity (counts of service use), and price,[9] with adjustment for age, sex, and health status. As shown in Figure 2-3, price and quantity are negatively correlated; spending is relatively uncorrelated with quantity, but highly correlated with price. This finding highlights the importance of further examining variation in commercial prices to understand its relationship to total commercial spending.

In a separate analysis, Harvard investigators disaggregated price into its subcomponents and examined variation in input prices and markups (defined as the difference between input and transaction "output" prices). Harvard reports that 70 percent of variation in total commercial spending is attributable to price markups, most likely reflecting the varying market

---

[8]Note that this result differs from the finding in MedPAC's 2011 *Report to Congress: Regional Variation in Medicare Service Use*, which reports that input price adjustment decreased variation between metropolitan CBSAs in the 90th and 10th percentiles from 55 percent to 30 percent. Differences in the time period (MedPAC data are from 2006-2008), the data file used (MedPAC uses the beneficiary-level annual summary file [BASF] and inpatient claims), and especially in standardization methods could explain this discrepancy. Acumen used claim-level standardization for all Medicare Part A and B services, while MedPAC used claim-level standardization only for inpatient claims and the BASF for all other claims. In the BASF files, payment adjustments are based on the location of the beneficiary rather than the location of the provider. Acumen adjusted all Part A and B spending for the input price of the provider's location. Acumen then aggregated each individual's total price-adjusted spending and assigned this amount to the location (i.e., HRR) in which the individual resided.

[9]Refer to the Harvard report for detail on the methodology of the price calculation (Harvard University, 2012).

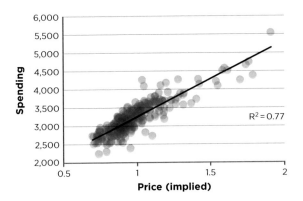

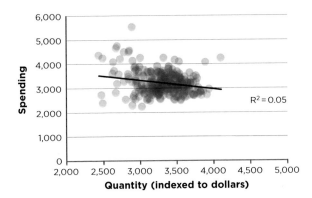

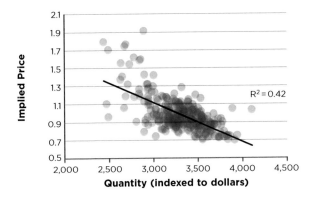

FIGURE 2-3 Relationships among spending, implied price and quantity, with adjustment for age, sex, and health status.

SOURCE: Harvard University, 2012.

TABLE 2-7
Relative Proportion of Spending Variation Due to Quantity (utilization), Markup, and Input Price, Decomposed by Service Type

	Quantity (%)	Markup (%)	Input-Price (%)
Total Medical Spending	16	70	14
Inpatient Spending	18	62	20
Outpatient Spending	21	70	9

SOURCE: Harvard University, 2012.

power of providers across HRRs (Harvard University, 2012).[10] As discussed earlier, variation in the utilization of health care services, particularly inpatient hospitalization and emergency department visits, does contribute to regional spending differences in the commercial population. As shown in Table 2-7, however, utilization and input prices have noticeably smaller effects than price markups on overall variation in commercial spending.

Conclusion 2.2. Variation in spending in the commercial insurance market is due mainly to differences in price markups by providers rather than to the differences in the utilization of health care services.

OTHER FACTORS ACCOUNTING FOR GEOGRAPHIC VARIATION

As noted in Chapter 1, reducing regional differences in health care spending and utilization is desirable only to the extent that the variation reflects system inefficiencies. A number of factors contribute to geographic variation, and while many of these factors have traditionally been classified as "acceptable" or "unacceptable," some sources of variation are ambiguous and do not fall neatly into either category. Area-level differences in factor prices (wage, rent, and other overhead costs) and in patient health status and demographic characteristics (e.g., age, gender) generally are considered to be acceptable sources of variation (American Hospital Association, 2011; Bernstein et al., 2011) because they are beyond the control of both providers and patients. By contrast, geographic variation in spend-

---

[10]It is widely believed that variation in prices for services delivered to commercially insured patients is driven by variation in provider market power. This belief has been difficult to confirm or refute empirically. It is not straightforward, for example, to define the boundaries for the relevant market; the relevant region for providing radiation therapy services differs from the region for acute cardiac care, for example, so a hospital may have a very large market share for one service and not for another. Consequently, market power may very well explain much of the variation in pricing for commercially insured patients, but appropriate empirical tests are difficult to implement.

ing is considered inappropriate or "unacceptable" when it is caused by or results in ineffective use of treatments, as by provider failure to adhere to established clinical practice guidelines, or when it reflects the market power of providers. As noted, not all causes of variation can be neatly classified. Variation stemming from differential patient preferences may potentially be acceptable, although more intensive treatment does not necessarily lead to higher-value care. Other demographic factors, such as race, represent a mix of acceptable and unacceptable causes of variation. If health needs vary by race across populations, it will be important to account for its effects. If race were responsible for preferences for care or discrimination, however, it would not be considered an acceptable source of variation in health care utilization. The literature shows a lack of consensus on a definitive framework for acceptable and unacceptable variation, and the interpretation of the association of such factors as patient preferences or race with variation is unclear.

A review of the literature on geographic variations reveals patient health status to be a key explanatory factor; however, estimates of its contribution vary greatly. Adjusting for health status has been shown to reduce variation in Medicare spending by 16 to 66 percent (CBO, 2008; Cutler and Sheiner, 1999).[11] A recent study found that health status, measured at the individual level, accounted for 18 percent of the geographic difference between the highest- and lowest-spending Medicare quintiles (Bernstein et al., 2011; Sutherland et al., 2009). The wide range of the explanatory effect of health status is due in general to differences across studies in the geographic unit of analysis and the risk adjustment methodology.

Health status risk scores typically are measured based on diagnosis codes recorded on Medicare claims. Because these codes differentiate only modestly among patients with the same diagnoses, they cannot perfectly capture true illness severity (Pine et al., 2007). Therefore, using such measures may fail to correct fully for differences in health status among areas. Moreover, risk adjustment using claims-based measures such as CMS's hierarchical condition category (HCC) codes may be subject to bias, as regions that have higher spending and greater intensity of practice appear to code more intensively, thus overstating beneficiaries' severity of illness (Song et al., 2010). As a result, at least some of the reduction in variation attribut-

---

[11]The 2008 Congressional Budget Office report states that previous work by MedPAC had concluded that 16 percent of variation in spending should be attributable to regional differences in beneficiary health status (CBO, 2008). This analysis was conducted at the state-level and weighted by population. The Cutler and Sheiner (1999) analysis, on the other hand, conducted at the HRR level with unweighted estimates, found that 66 percent of variation could be accounted for by differences in health status. It is unclear whether these studies used retrospective or prospective analysis. These differences in methodology can partially explain the large range of explanatory power attributable to health status (Manning et al., 2012).

able to health status using claims-based measures is an artifact of more aggressive surveillance and diagnosis by providers in higher-spending regions, although how important this bias is in attributing differences in spending among regions to differences in health status has not been quantified.

Adjusting for patient burden of illness using more complete measures of health status naturally accounts for a greater portion of unexplained geographic variation in Medicare spending. A recent study found that using progressively better and more comprehensive measures of health status reduced unexplained variation by 21-33 percent (Zuckerman et al., 2010). A separate evaluation of Medicare Part D (prescription drug) risk adjustment methodology found that incorporating information on prior-year drug use, cost, or both into CMS's prescription drug HCC (RxHCC) greatly improved the variation explained (Hsu et al., 2009). For example, using a CMS-HCC summary score explained 10 percent of variation in Medicare drug spending, while including more detailed information and using 184 HCC indicators explained 17 percent. Respecting practical limitations, ideally health status measures based on claims data should be enhanced with important behavioral and clinical data on Medicare and commercially insured beneficiaries.

Previous studies have found that demographic variables such as age, sex, race, ethnicity, and income are common confounders of individual patient health (Adler and Newman, 2002; Case and Deaton, 2005; DeNavas-Walt et al., 2009; Farley, 1985). As discussed earlier, differences in the regional distribution of these factors may subsequently influence aggregated, area-level health care spending and utilization. Although the age and sex composition of Medicare beneficiaries is generally similar across large geographic areas, race and income patterns are more heterogeneous (Baicker, 2004; Baicker et al., 2005). In 2004, approximately 80 percent of Hispanics in the United States lived in 9 states, while 60 percent of all African Americans were concentrated in 10 states (American Hospital Association, 2009). Furthermore, disease burden and associated medical spending vary among different races; for example, one study found that African American Medicare beneficiaries had higher health care spending than non-Hispanic white beneficiaries (Baicker et al., 2004). It is important to note that demographic variables, including gender, age, race/ethnicity, and income, continue to serve as proxies for other, unmeasured behavioral and socioeconomic predictors of health status. Although there is some heterogeneity in the distribution of demographic variables throughout the United States, they may be close enough to uniform that they do not explain variation at the area level, particularly after variation attributable to patient health status is accounted for.

To date, few studies have investigated the degree to which the type and benefit generosity of insurance plans contribute to measures of geographic variation in health care spending and utilization. The benefits associated with specific insurance plans, including deductibles, copayments, and other internal limits, can affect how much health care is consumed, as well as what health care is provided (Finkelstein et al., 2012; Newhouse and Insurance Experiment Group, 1993). In comparing spending by payer type, a recent study found more variation in hospitalizations across metropolitan areas for populations with unmanaged care than for those enrolled in an HMO (Baker et al., 2010). The committee's empirical analyses of Medicare and commercial spending, utilization, and quality adjusted for regional differences attributable to these predictors, as discussed in the following sections and in Chapter 4.

In addition to population and patient characteristics, geographic variation in health care spending and utilization may be influenced by a host of local and regional market factors, such as the supply of providers and medical services, the percentage composition of the insured population, and provider and payer competition (Baicker et al., 2004; Fisher et al., 2003a; Reschovsky et al., 2011; Welch et al., 1993; Wennberg and Cooper, 1999). The types of providers within a defined area (HRR, state, other definitions) may affect variation in health care spending; recent studies have found a correlation between a higher percentage of primary care physicians and lower spending per beneficiary within a region (Baicker et al., 2005; Chernew et al., 2009). Greater hospital capacity within regions, which translates to a higher ratio of beds to per capita population, is correlated with higher health care utilization, particularly affecting rates of inpatient hospital admission (Wennberg et al., 2004). Although the supply of physicians and hospitals is correlated with health care spending and utilization, there may not necessarily be a causal connection, as variables such as physician supply and hospital capacity are endogenous in nature.

EMPIRICAL EVALUATION OF PREDICTORS OF VARIATION

The committee's commissioned analyses complement the existing literature, evaluating the role of patient-, payer-, and market-level factors on geographic variation in health care spending and utilization. The subcontractors conducted multiple ordinary least squares (OLS) regression analyses at the HSA, HRR, and metropolitan CBSA levels, controlling for "clusters" of established predictors.[12] In selecting a baseline case model (Cluster 2), the committee adjusted for "acceptable" and expected sources of geographic variation, such patient health status, age, and sex. The baseline model does not adjust for other, ambiguous demographic factors,

---

[12]See Table 2-8 and Appendix D for a complete list of predictors and regression model specifications.

such as race and income, as these variables are distributed heterogeneously across regions, suggesting that some areas may have greater access to or can afford better health care. The baseline case model also does not adjust for endogenous factors such as market supply variables, which, like race and income, are considered by some to be "unacceptable" sources of variation.

Table 2-8 shows how the HRR-level distribution of the highest-spending (90th percentile) and lowest-spending (10th percentile) quintiles changes with adjustment for regional differences in predictors. Results indicate that adjusting for age and sex (Cluster 1) has a negligible effect on geographic variation in Medicare spending. Beneficiary health status (Cluster 2), when measured using diagnoses recorded on claims, substantially reduces variation between high- and low-spending regions across both Medicare and commercial payers.[13] This suggests that diagnoses recorded on claims are systematically different across HRRs. Therefore, the base case adjustments (Cluster 2) account for much of the variation in input-price-adjusted spending.

Figure 2-4 illustrates the change in geographic variation in Medicare input-price-adjusted spending after adjustment for age, sex, and health status predictors (Control and Cluster 2 in Table 2-8). Each bar represents the number of people in HRRs with a given spending level. For example, the far left bar in the top histogram indicates that around a million people live in HRRs with Medicare spending under $700. The lower histogram is adjusted for age, sex, and health status, whereas the upper one is not. As indicated by the narrowed distribution of the 90th to the 10th percentile ratios (1.44 to 1.23) in the lower histogram, a greater number of HRRs (weighted by beneficiary months) fall in the middle range of Medicare spending when age, sex, and health status are taken into account.

Results of the Cluster 3 and 4 regressions in Table 2-8 demonstrate that when health status is excluded from the model, other demographic variables, such as race or income, provide little explanatory power.[14] Cluster 5 results confirm that race and income have a trivial effect on reducing variation once beneficiary health status is included in the model. Insurance and employer characteristics (Cluster 6) also explain some regional variation in the commercially insured population.

Comparing the results of Clusters 2 and 8 shows that once age, sex,

---

[13]In the Harvard MarketScan regression analysis, spending variation is reduced most substantially with adjustment for age and sex (Cluster 1), and health status (Cluster 2) appears not to provide additional explanatory power. As age and sex are common confounders for health status, however, this may be a result of measurement issues in the data. The combined effect of demographic variables and health status on variation is considerably large.

[14]Race and income variables have a slightly greater effect in the MarketScan population than in the Medicare and OptumInsight populations. This difference in results may be attributed to varying sample sizes in each HRR across the different databases.

TABLE 2-8
Ratios of 90th to 10th Percentile HRR-Level Input-Price-Adjusted Spending Across Payers When Adjusted for "Clusters" of Predictors

Cluster	Ratio: Medicare	Ratio: Commercial 1 (OptumInsight)	Ratio: Commercial 2 (MarketScan)
Control: *Adjusted for Year and Partial-Year Enrollment Only*	1.44	1.43	1.33
Cluster 1: *Adjusted for Control + Age + Sex + Age–Sex Interaction*	1.44	1.43	1.26
Cluster 2: *Adjusted for Cluster 1 + Health Status[a]*	1.23	1.37	1.28
Cluster 3: *Adjusted for Cluster 1 + Race*	1.40	1.43	1.24
Cluster 4: *Adjusted for Cluster 1 + Income*	1.41	1.40	1.26
Cluster 5: *Adjusted for Cluster 1 + Race + Income + Health Status*	1.25	1.42	1.27
Cluster 6: *Adjusted for Cluster 1 + Employer/Insurance Predictors[b]*	*	1.39	1.30
Cluster 7: *Adjusted for Cluster 1 + Market-Level Predictors[c]*	1.44	**	1.26
Cluster 8[d,e]: *Adjusted for Cluster 5 + Employer/Insurance Predictors + Market-Level Predictors*	1.25	**	1.28
Cluster 9[e]: *Adjusted for Cluster 5 + Employer/Insurance Predictors + Reduced Set of Market-Level Predictors*	1.25	**	1.27
Cluster 10[e]: *Adjusted for Cluster 1 + Medicare-Specific Variables[d]*	1.25	***	***

[a]The analysis uses CMS's 2008 definition of hierarchical condition categories (HCCs) as an indicator of health status.

[b]Employer and insurance characteristics include the following variables: benefit generosity, payer/plan type, plan size (OptumInsight only), and data source (MarketScan only).

[c]Market-level predictors include the following variables: hospital competition, % uninsured population, supply of medical services, malpractice environmental risk, physician composition, access to care, payer mix, Medicaid penetration, health professional mix, supplemental Medicare insurance.

[d]Cluster 8 combines all predictors used in Clusters 1-7. These include demographic variables (age, gender, race, income), health status, employer and insurance characteristics, and market-level factors. In addition to the specified predictors, this model also includes dummy indicators for institutional status, dual-enrollment status, and supplemental Medicare insurance.

[e]See Appendix D for complete model specifications for the Medicare analysis.

*This regression was conducted using commercial insurance data only, as it was not applicable to the Medicare analysis.

**The methodology used to conduct the OptumInsight market-level analysis differed substantially from that of the other analyses, making the results noncomparable across subcontractors. Refer to Lewin's report for complete findings (The Lewin Group, 2013).

***This regression specification was limited to the Medicare analysis.

SOURCE: Committee analysis of subcontractor data.

and health status are accounted for, the full set of market variables does not reduce variation in either the Medicare or commercially insured population. Even after adjustment for all predictors measurable within the data used for these analyses and supported by the literature (demographic factors, health status, insurance and employer characteristics, and market-level covariates), a substantial amount of variation remains unexplained. The degree to which this variation represents "unacceptable" variation or inefficiency rather than potentially "acceptable" variation due to factors not measured by the data (such as patient preferences and health behaviors) is unknown.

Results differ for the commercial population. Much of the variation in spending in that population is attributable to differential markups, which are not present in the Medicare population since CMS sets a take-it-or-leave-it price. Not surprisingly, market factors play a role in explaining the variation attributable to these markups; accounting for them reduces the variation in the markups by 27 percent. Because of the negative correlation between markups and quantity (utilization) of health care, however, market factors and spending show little correlation (see Table 2-8).

Moreover, the results of PHE's analysis of variation in total, input-price-adjusted health care spending attributable to known predictors, displayed in Table 2-9, reveal a pattern similar to that of Medicare- and commercial-only spending. The drop in the 90th to 10th percentile ratio between the Control and Cluster 2 regression models suggests that age, sex, and health status of beneficiaries account for a substantial portion of variation across HRRs. Factors such as race, income, and market variables do not provide additional explanatory power once age, sex, and health status are included in the model. Moreover, unexplained variation remains that may be a result of unobservable, unmeasured acceptable factors or unacceptable inefficiencies.

These analyses were limited to predictors measurable with claims data. As a result, the regional variation attributable to patient preferences and access to care or to differences in physician discretion and practice patterns, for example, could not be measured.

Patient access to care has been shown to influence Medicare spending and utilization. Fisher and Wennberg (2003) conclude that HRRs that provide lower access to care, with long waiting times for office or emergency department visits, also tend to have higher expenditures (Fisher and Wennberg, 2003). Although patient access to medical care varies across regions in the United States as the result of a number of socioeconomic factors (Fiscella et al., 2000), it appears to have little impact on patients' perceived quality of care (Fowler et al., 2008; Radley, 2012).

It is unclear what proportion of overall variation can be accounted for by regional variation in patient preferences, a variable that is challenging to measure with accuracy. Some studies have found an association between

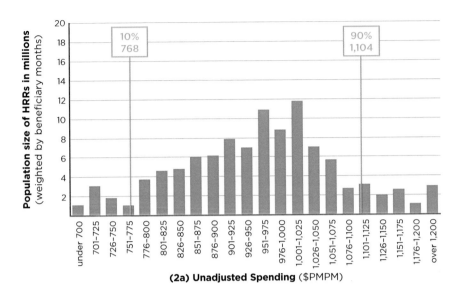

(2a) Unadjusted Spending ($PMPM)

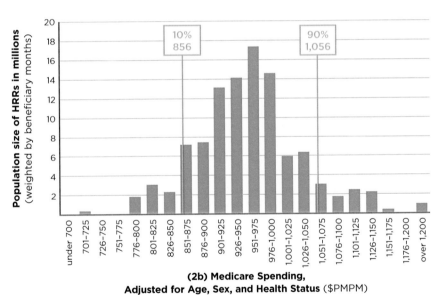

(2b) Medicare Spending,
Adjusted for Age, Sex, and Health Status ($PMPM)

FIGURE 2-4 Number of Medicare beneficiaries in hospital referral regions (HRRs) in 22 categories of monthly per capita spending, with input-price adjustment alone (2a—top) and with input-price adjustment plus adjustment for age, sex, and health status (2b—bottom).

NOTE: Medicare spending in both 2a and 2b have been adjusted for regional difference in input price. PMPM = per patient per month.

SOURCE: Developed by the committee and IOM staff based on data from Acumen Medicare analysis.

TABLE 2-9

Ratios of 90th to 10th Percentile HRR-Level Input-Price-Adjusted Total Health Care Spending When Adjusted for Selected "Clusters" of Predictors

Cluster	Ratio: Total Spending
Control: *No adjustments*	1.48
Cluster 2: *Adjusted for Partial Year Enrollment + Age + Sex + Age–Sex Interaction + Health Status*	1.32
Cluster 3: *Adjusted for Cluster 2 + Race*	1.31
Cluster 4: *Adjusted for Cluster 2 + Income*	1.31
Cluster 5: *Adjusted for Cluster 2 + Race + Income*	1.31
Cluster 7: *Adjusted for Cluster 2 + Market Variables[a]*	1.32
Cluster 9[e]: *Adjusted for Cluster 5 + Market Variables[a]*	1.29

[a]Precision Health Economics selected a reduced set of market-level variables from those originally provided in the Acumen, Lewin, and Harvard reports on Medicare and commercial data according to several criteria: policy relevance, consistency of measurement, lack of redundancy, and effect size of predictors in the commissioned analyses,. The following market-level covariates were used in this analysis: specialists per 1,000, beds per 1,000, Herfindahl–Hirschman Index (HHI) distribution of beds, % health maintenance organization (HMO) population, % uninsured population, total population, teaching hospital indicator, malpractice geographic practice cost index (GPCI) indicator.

SOURCE: PHE, 2013.

variation in patient preferences and geographic variation in health care utilization, while others have established that patient preferences account for little regional variation in health care spending (Anthony et al., 2009; Barnato et al., 2007).

The role of physicians in explaining regional variation is better established. Numerous studies have found that differences in provider practice patterns can explain a substantial portion of geographic variation (Baicker, 2004; MedPAC, 2008; Sirovich et al., 2005, 2008). In fact, physician decision making can account for more than half the variation in spending on end-of-life care across geographic areas (Cutler et al., 2013). Specifically, differences in physicians' beliefs about the efficacy of certain discretionary treatments explain the largest proportion of regional variation, followed by physicians' views on organizational factors (pressure to accommodate other providers or patients). The associated analysis found that financial incentives do not play a role. The investigators note that provider beliefs often are not correlated with current medical professional guidelines in the United States. This suggested lack of application of evidence-based treatment that promotes high value may represent waste or inefficiency within the health care system.

The subcontractors' analyses do not distinguish between "acceptable" and "unacceptable" sources of variation. The residual variation unaccounted for here may have a causal connection with unobservable factors, such as patient preferences, unmeasured regional differences in health status, market characteristics, or discretionary provision of inefficient care. Some variation is driven by policies specific to certain health care services or is attributable to unique regional factors, such as Medicare fraud. By definition, it is impossible to infer how much variation is attributable to each of these unmeasured factors. However, the robust presence of sizable residual variation in the use of health care services, even as more and more causes of "acceptable" variation are measured, creates a presumption that inefficiency may be one of the potential causes of variation.

Conclusion 2.3. The committee's empirical analysis revealed that after accounting for differences in age, sex, and health status, geographic variation is not further explained by other beneficiary demographic factors, insurance plan factors, or market-level characteristics. In fact, after controlling for all factors measurable within the data used for this analysis, a large amount of variation remains unexplained.

INFLUENCE OF POST-ACUTE CARE SERVICES ON REGIONAL VARIATION IN MEDICARE

To determine the extent to which variation in particular health care services contributes to total variation in Medicare expenditures, the committee disaggregated price-standardized, risk-adjusted Medicare spending into seven types of services: (1) acute (inpatient) care, (2) post-acute care, (3) prescription drugs, (4) diagnostics, (5) procedures, (6) emergency department visits, and (7) other.[15] Results of the subcontractors' analyses suggest that utilization of post-acute care services is a key driver of HRR-level variation in Medicare spending, with most of the remaining variation stemming from use of inpatient services. Post-acute care includes a wide

---

[15]"Acute care" includes inpatient claims at acute hospitals and Medicare Part B claims when the place of service is an inpatient hospital; it excludes claims from psychiatric and rehabilitation facilities. "Post-acute care" includes home health care, skilled nursing care, hospice care, rehabilitation, and long-term care hospitals. "Prescription drugs" includes Medicare Parts B and D. "Diagnostics" includes outpatient physician visits and imaging. "Other" denotes all claims not included in the first six categories.

range of services designed to treat beneficiaries following discharge from an acute care hospital setting. A recent study reports that in 2002, approximately one-third of Medicare beneficiaries who received treatment at acute care hospitals also used post-acute care services (American Hospital Association, 2009).

The key role played by post-acute care services can be clearly seen in Figures 2-5a through 2-5h, a series of charts in which the horizontal axis represents HRRs ordered from left to right by total per-member-per-month, input-price-adjusted spending (a measure of utilization) between 2007 and 2009 for Medicare Parts A and B. Thus in each graph, the lowest total use area (Rochester, New York) is the left-most bar, and the highest total use area (Miami, Florida) is the right-most. The vertical axis represents the deviation of input-price-adjusted spending (utilization) in a particular HRR from the national mean utilization for the type of service shown after adjustment for patient demographics and health status (see the note to the figures). In other words, the residuals represent unexplained variation. Figure 2-5a shows the total Medicare utilization across HRRs that remains unexplained after adjustment for input prices, demographics, and health status, while Figures 2-5b through 2-5h display the unexplained variation in utilization in specific service categories only. These residual charts suggest that variation in post-acute care utilization accounts for a large portion of the unexplained variation in total utilization. Areas to the far left in Figure 2-5a have utilization roughly $50 to $150 below the adjusted national mean, whereas those on the far right have utilization roughly $100 to $200 above the adjusted national mean. In fact, as Table 2-10 indicates, if there were no variation in post-acute care spending, the variation in total spending would fall by 73 percent. Miami is an outlier, which the committee addresses in greater detail below.

Almost all of the remaining variation is accounted for by variation in acute (inpatient) care utilization (see Figure 2-5c). If there were no variation in acute care spending but the variation in post-acute care spending were unchanged, the variation in total spending would fall by 27 percent. Finally, if there were no variation in either acute or post-acute care spending, variation in total spending would fall by 89 percent (see Table 2-10). Thus, the remaining services shown (e.g., diagnostic, which includes outpatient physician services; emergency department/ambulance service; and prescription drugs) play a small role in variation in Medicare spending.

As discussed previously, the subcontractors' findings are consistent with those of MedPAC's 2011 report to Congress, which reveal that utilization of post-acute care and acute (inpatient) care accounts for the greatest variability in Medicare spending (MedPAC, 2011). Prior studies have noted that variation in the use of post-acute care is influenced not only by demographic and clinical factors but also by a number of nonclinical predictors, including "variation in provider practice patterns, differences in local regulatory practices, and supply of [post-acute care] services" (Kane et al., 2002). Availability of and access to different types of post-acute care services also were found to be a determinant of utilization (Buntin et al., 2005). Although the subcontractors' post-acute care analyses did not adjust for market factors (for example, supply of post-acute care facilities and beds), previous results of regression modeling (presented in Table 2-8) demonstrate that, after accounting for age, sex, and health status, market factors do not provide additional explanatory power.

The committee noted that certain geographic areas spent considerably more than others for specific high-margin goods and services (e.g., home health care and durable medical equipment). The geographic variation in home health care spending may be partially accounted for by the variation in beneficiary and provider adherence to program standards (MedPAC, 2012). The comprehensive coverage criteria allow beneficiaries to receive an unlimited number of home health care episodes once they qualify, and provide no incentives for either beneficiaries or physicians to consider alternative treatments. Some evidence also suggests that providers do not consistently follow Medicare's standards in designing treatment. Although these differences in practice patterns explain some variation in home health care, the literature suggests that large deviations from the national average in spending and utilization in some areas may be an indication of fraud (Bernstein et al., 2011; MedPAC, 2009). In fact, the U.S. Office of the Inspector General (OIG) identified certain geographic areas in Florida, Illinois, Louisiana, Michigan, New York, and Texas as high-risk for Medicare fraud (OIG, 2012). For example, Table 2-11 shows data from MedPAC on spending on home health care and durable medical equipment in the four southernmost Florida counties in 2006 and 2008 (MedPAC, 2011). Miami-Dade County is a clear outlier, with per capita spending substantially greater than that of other nearby areas. Additionally, "in 2009, OIG found that Miami-Dade County, Florida, accounted for more home health outlier payments in 2008 than the rest of the Nation combined and that 67 percent of home health agencies that received outlier payments greater than $1 million were located in Miami-Dade County" (OIG, 2012, p. 9).

As described earlier, not all sources of variation can be measured, and variation in spending attributable to geographic variation in fraud is one such source. Although the amount of annual Medicare spending due to fraud is, by definition, unknown (Goldman, 2012), recent estimates indicate that Medicare and Medicaid paid as much as $98 billion in fraudulent and abusive charges in 2011 (Berwick and Hackbarth, 2012). Because fraud represents care that is never delivered to a patient and consequently cannot improve health, a geographic payment adjustment based on area-level performance would penalize areas with above-average fraud. Yet, if such

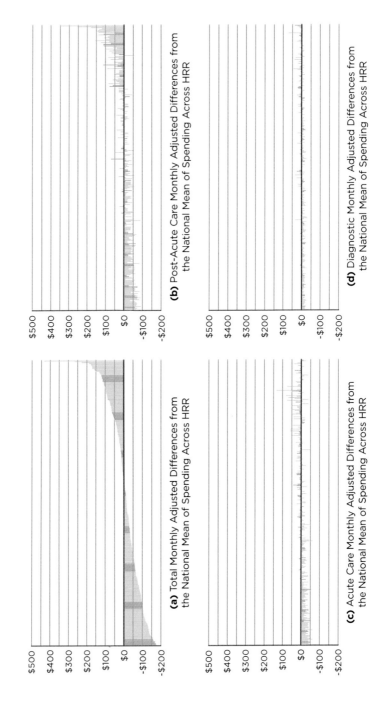

(a) Total Monthly Adjusted Differences from the National Mean of Spending Across HRR

(b) Post-Acute Care Monthly Adjusted Differences from the National Mean of Spending Across HRR

(c) Acute Care Monthly Adjusted Differences from the National Mean of Spending Across HRR

(d) Diagnostic Monthly Adjusted Differences from the National Mean of Spending Across HRR

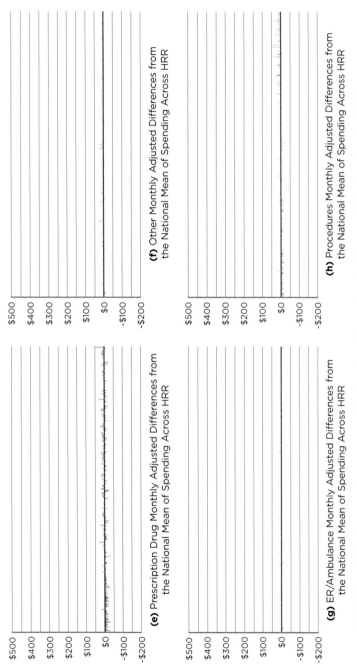

$500
$400
$300
$200
$100
$0
-$100
-$200

(e) Prescription Drug Monthly Adjusted Differences from the National Mean of Spending Across HRR

$500
$400
$300
$200
$100
$0
-$100
-$200

(f) Other Monthly Adjusted Differences from the National Mean of Spending Across HRR

$500
$400
$300
$200
$100
$0
-$100
-$200

(g) ER/Ambulance Monthly Adjusted Differences from the National Mean of Spending Across HRR

$500
$400
$300
$200
$100
$0
-$100
-$200

(h) Procedures Monthly Adjusted Differences from the National Mean of Spending Across HRR

FIGURE 2-5a-h Medicare service category utilization (monthly cost residual) by hospital referral region (HRR).

NOTE: In this analysis, utilization is measured as the the total per-member-per-month input-price-adjusted cost (the dollar amounts shown at the left of each figure). The predictor variables include beneficiary age; sex; age-sex interaction; race; health status coded by hierarchical condition category; partial-year enrollment; and indicators for supplemental Medicare insurance, institutionalization status, new enrollee status (prior-year diagnoses are not available for them), dual-enrollment status, and year of analysis (2007, 2008, 2009). Selected results displaying the residual total post-acute and acute care costs for all 306 HRRs are available in Appendix G.

SOURCE: Acumen, LLC, 2013a.

TABLE 2-10
Proportion of Variance Attributable to Each Medicare Service Category

	Adjusted Total Medicare Spending	
	Remaining Variance	Reduction in Variance (%)*
Variation in Total Medicare Spending	6,974	—
If No Variation in Post-Acute Care Only	1,864	73
If No Variation in Acute Care Only	5,085	27
If No Variation in Either Post-Acute or Acute	780	89
If No Variation in Prescription Drugs	6,374	9
If No Variation in Diagnostic Tests	5,986	14
If No Variation in Procedures	6,020	14
If No Variation in Emergency Department Visits/Ambulance Use	6,972	0
If No Variation in Other	6,882	1

NOTE: Total Medicare spending and each component are input-price- and risk-adjusted. Each row shows the reduction in variance from eliminating only the variation in that service, with the exception of the acute and post-acute care rows.

*The individual reductions sum to more than 100 percent because of covariance terms.

SOURCE: Committee analysis of Medicare data.

counties were penalized for being low-value, all legitimate providers in those counties would bear the consequences.

> *Conclusion 2.4. Variation in total Medicare spending across geographic areas is driven largely by variation in the utilization of post-acute care services, and to a lesser extent by variation in the utilization of acute care services.*

LIMITATIONS OF EFFORTS TO MEASURE VARIATION IN QUALITY

Health care quality "composite measures" allow measurement of multiple aspects of quality by collapsing individual measures to create a single score (NQF, 2009). Composite quality indicators, developed and maintained by the Agency for Healthcare Research and Quality (AHRQ), are based largely on administrative data (billing- or claims-related information), with inclusion and exclusion criteria being based on diagnosis or procedure codes. The committee's commissioned analyses evaluated quality

TABLE 2-11
Wide Variation in Spending for Durable Medical Equipment and Home Health Care in Contiguous Florida Counties

Area	DME Spending per Capita ($)		Home Health Care Spending per Capita ($)	
	2006	2008	2006	2008
South Florida County				
Broward	394	321	1,002	1,390
Collier	207	202	305	395
Miami-Dade	2,043	828	2,591	5,318
Monroe	237	210	237	334
National	263	282	382	488

NOTES: DME = durable medical equipment. Spending data are annualized for beneficiaries with either Part A or Part B coverage for at least 1 month during 2006. The results are not adjusted for differences in beneficiaries' health status or prices. In March 2007, the U.S. Department of Justice, the U.S. Attorney's Office for the Southern District of Florida, the Department of Health and Human Services (HHS), OIG, and state and local law enforcement launched the Medicare Fraud Strike Force in South Florida. In its early stages, the task force targeted fraud in HIV infusion therapy and DME (DOJ, 2013; Katz, 2012), which may explain the significant drop in DME spending observed between 2006 and 2008 in Miami-Dade County.

SOURCE: MedPAC, 2011, p. 11.

of care using both individual measures and the following nationally established composite quality indicators:

- *Prevention Quality Indicator (PQI) #90*: Reflects the quality of ambulatory care in preventing medical complications for both acute and chronic illness.
- *Inpatient Quality Composite Indicator (IQI) #91*: Reflects the quality of care delivered in an inpatient hospital setting, and includes mortality indicators, as well as procedures for which there is a question of inefficient use.
- *Patient Safety Indicator (PSI) #90*: Reflects the quality of care within a hospital, particularly as it relates to potentially preventable surgical complications or iatrogenic events.
- *Pediatric Quality Indicator (PDI) #19*: Reflects the quality of care among the pediatric population.

Although these national quality indicators represent the "current state of the art in assessing the health care system as a whole," performance measures based on administrative data have a number of limitations (Farquhar, 2008). For instance, the complex association between preventive care in an outpatient setting (PQI) and beneficiary socioeconomic status often complicates an assessment of regional variation because such factors as patient access to care, patient preferences, and other unmeasured barriers in traditionally underserved populations cannot be accounted for (AHRQ, 2007a). Measurement of preventable complications (PSI) may be limited by inaccuracies within the underlying data, as providers who fear negative consequences are unlikely to maintain a thorough record of preventable complications in their patients (AHRQ, 2007b). As discussed previously, studies have established differences in coding practices among physicians, as well as among hospitals, making a fair comparison of hospitals (based on IQI) difficult. Moreover, administrative data are "clinically vague," as the same diagnosis code may be applied to a heterogeneous pool of clinical states. As a result, risk adjustment of administrative claims is likely to be imperfect, and this may affect the measurement of quality.

As discussed earlier, although the subcontractors' regression analyses risk adjust for certain known predictors (including age, sex, and health status), a number of unmeasured factors may account for variation in quality across areas.[16] This report does not quantify the amount of geographic variation in health care quality as it does for spending and utilization because of limitations in the measurement of quality composites and the underlying data. All of the commissioned analyses report on two measures of health care quality—PSI and PQI. The Harvard and Lewin analyses each include quality measures that are "rare" among commercially insured populations. Although previous research has noted some differences in quality patterns across the United States (MedPAC, 2003), greater emphasis has been placed on studying relationships among quality, overall spending, and "high value." In Chapter 4, the committee evaluates the use of a geographically based value index and further explores the empirical interrelationships among quality of care and health care spending and utilization across Medicare and private payers.

RESEARCH AGENDA

This study represents the largest-scale analysis of geographic variation in health care spending in the United States, covering Medicare and representative private payer populations. The availability of and access to CMS's complete Medicare (Parts A, B, C, and D) claims database were instrumental to the successful completion of this research. As discussed previously, however, the lack of access to encounter claims information for Medicare

---

[16]The subcontractors all followed AHRQ guidelines but used varying methodologies to calculate quality composites. Refer to Appendix C for a brief summary and to the Acumen, Lewin, and Harvard reports for complete details. (Subcontractor reports can be accessed through the Institute of Medicine website at http://www.iom.edu/geovariationmaterials.)

and Medicaid managed care enrollees during the 2007-2009 period limits the generalizability of the study findings. Although CMS has in recent years made an effort to improve and simplify the process of obtaining historical data, significant operational, procedural, and financial barriers continue to exist. Congress could help remove these barriers by supporting CMS's efforts to expand the availability of Medicare and Medicaid data for research purposes, with particular emphasis on releasing previously unavailable or limited Medicare Part C and D data. For its part, CMS could use its existing authority to broaden data access for the purposes of primary research and evaluation while safeguarding patient privacy and maintaining standards established by the Social Security Act, the Health Insurance Portability and Accountability Act (HIPAA) Privacy Rule, the Privacy Act of 1974, and the Federal Information Security and Management Act of 2002 (FISMA).

As noted in earlier sections of this chapter, current understanding of health care utilization and quality is limited as it depends on information available in administrative (claims and billing) data, which do not capture the extent or severity of a patient's illness. CMS could enrich claims databases by better adjusting for population health and could assist in the creation of more accurate quality measures by creating a platform for clinical and behavioral information (e.g., electronic medical records).

More research on health care outcomes and quality is needed, particularly for commercially insured populations. To date, many nationally established quality composite measures have been designed to measure process and outcomes in the Medicare population and are not necessarily applicable to privately insured beneficiaries. Although in its estimate of total health care spending in the United States, PHE attempted to include estimates from Medicare, Medicaid, and commercial payers, as well as the uninsured, the generalizability of this analysis is limited. Further research on this topic is needed and would benefit from the availabilty of a national-level all-payer database. Moreover, combined use of Medicare and private administrative or claims data would allow for more accurate measurement of provider performance and quality of care. Collaboration between CMS and private payers would be an important first step toward creating an enriched national data source.

> **RECOMMENDATION 1: Congress should encourage the Centers for Medicare & Medicaid Services (CMS), and provide the necessary resources, to make accessing Medicare and Medicaid data easier for research purposes. CMS should collaborate with private insurers to collect, integrate, and analyze standardized data on spending, as well as clinical and behavioral health outcomes, to enable more extensive comparisons of payments and quality and evaluation of value-based payment models across payers.**

REFERENCES

Acumen, LLC. 2009. *Revision of Medicare Wage Index—Final Report: Part I.* Burlingame, CA.

————. 2013a. *Geographic variation in spending, utilization and quality: Medicare and Medicaid beneficiaries.* Washington, DC: Institute of Medicine.

————. 2013b. *IOM study of geographic variation: Growth analysis.* Washington, DC: Institute of Medicine.

Adler, N. E., and K. Newman. 2002. Socioeconomic disparities in health: Pathways and policies. *Health Affairs* 21(2):60-76.

AHRQ (Agency for Healthcare Research and Quality). 2007a. *AHRQ guide to prevention quality indicators: Hospital admission for ambulatory sensitive conditions.* Edited by U.S. Department of Health and Human Services. Rockville, MD.

————. 2007b. *AHRQ guide to patient safety indicators.* Edited by U.S. Department of Health and Human Services. Rockville, MD, March 12.

American Hospital Association. 2009. Geographic variation in health care spending: A closer look. In *Trend Watch.* Washington, DC: American Hospital Association.

————. 2011. *Report of the Task Force on Variation in Health Care Spending.* Washington, DC: American Hospital Association.

Anthony, D. L., M. B. Herndon, P. M. Gallagher, A. E. Barnato, J. P. Bynum, D. J. Gottlieb, E. S. Fisher, and J. S. Skinner. 2009. How much do patients' preferences contribute to resource use? *Health Affairs* 28(3):864-873.

ASPE (Assistant Secretary for Planning and Evaluation). 2011. Overview of the uninsured in the United States: A summary of the 2011 current population survey. *ASPE Issue Brief.* http://aspe.hhs.gov/health/reports/2011/cpshealthins2011/ib.shtml (accessed July 18, 2013).

Autor, D., A. Chandra, and M. Duggan. 2011. *Public health expenditures on the working age disabled: Assessing Medicare: Public health expenditures on the working age disabled: Assessing Medicare.* Cambridge, MA: National Bureau of Economic Research.

Baicker, K., and A. Chandra. 2004. Medicare spending, the physician workforce, and beneficiaries' quality of care. *Health Affairs* Supplemental Web Exclusives W4-184-97.

Baicker, K., A. Chandra, J. S. Skinner, and J. E. Wennberg. 2004. Who you are and where you live: How race and geography affect the treatment of Medicare beneficiaries. *Health Affairs* Supplemental Variation 33-44.

Baicker, K., A. Chandra, and J. S. Skinner. 2005. Geographic variation in health care and the problem of measuring racial disparities. *Perspectives in Biology and Medicine* 48(Suppl. 1):S42-S53.

Baker, L. C., M. K. Bundorf, and D. P. Kessler. 2010. HMO coverage reduces variations in the use of health care among patients under age sixty-five. *Health Affairs* 29(11):2068-2074.

Barnato, A. E., M. B. Herndon, D. L. Anthony, P. M. Gallagher, J. S. Skinner, J. P. Bynum, and E. S. Fisher. 2007. Are regional variations in end-of-life care intensity explained by patient preferences? A study of the US Medicare population. *Medical Care* 45(5):386-393.

Bernstein, J., J. D. Reschovsky, and C. White. 2011. *Geographic variation in health care: Changing policy directions.* Washington, DC: National Institute for Health Care Reform.

Berwick, D. M., and A. D. Hackbarth. 2012. Eliminating waste in U.S. health care. *Journal of the American Medical Association* 307(14):1513-1516.

Buntin, M. B., A. D. Garten, S. Paddock, D. Saliba, M. Totten, and J. J. Escarce. 2005. How much is postacute care use affected by its availability? *Health Services Research* 40(2):413-434.

Case, A., and A. S. Deaton. 2005. Broken down by work and sex: How our health declines. In *Analyses in the economics of aging*. Chicago, IL: University of Chicago Press. Pp. 185-212.

CBO (Congressional Budget Office). 2008. *Geographic variation in health care spending*. Washington, DC: Congress of the United States, CBO.

Chernew, M. E., L. Sabik, A. Chandra, and J. P. Newhouse. 2009. Would having more primary care doctors cut health spending growth? *Health Affairs (Millwood)* 28(5):1327-1335.

Chernew, M. E., L. M. Sabik, A. Chandra, T. B. Gibson, and J. P. Newhouse. 2010. Geographic correlation between large-firm commercial spending and Medicare spending. *American Journal of Managed Care* 16(2):131-138.

CMS (Centers for Medicare & Medicaid Services). 2012. *Wage index*. http://www.cms.gov/Medicare/Medicare-Fee-for-Service-Payment/AcuteInpatientPPS/wageindex.html (accessed March 29, 2013).

Cummins, R. O. 1993. Emergency medical services and sudden cardiac arrest: The "chain of survival" concept. *Annual Review of Public Health* 14(1):313-333.

Cunningham, P. J. 2006. What accounts for differences in the use of hospital emergency departments across U.S. communities? *Health Affairs (Millwood)* 25(5):w324-w336.

Cutler, D. M., and L. Sheiner. 1999. The geography of Medicare. *American Economic Review* 89(2):228-233.

Cutler, D., J. Skinner, D. Stern, and D. Wennberg. 2013. *Physician beliefs and patient preferences: A new look at regional variation in spending*. https://www.lafollette.wisc.edu/research/health_economics/Stern.pdf (accessed July 18, 2013).

Dartmouth Institute for Health Policy and Clinical Practice. 2013. *The Dartmouth Atlas of Health Care*. http://www.dartmouthatlas.org (accessed July 18, 2013).

DeNavas-Walt, C., B. D. Proctor, and J. C. Smith. 2009. *Income, poverty, and health insurance coverage in the United States: 2009*. Washington, DC: U.S. Census Bureau.

DOJ (Department of Justice). 2013. *Health care fraud and abuse control program: Annual report for fiscal year 2012*. Washington, DC.

Donohue, J. M., N. E. Morden, W. F. Gellad, J. P. Bynum, W. Zhou, J. T. Hanlon, and J. Skinner. 2012. Sources of regional variation in Medicare Part D drug spending. *New England Journal of Medicine* 366(6):530-538.

Dunn, A., A. H. Shapiro, and E. Liebman. 2012. *Geographic variation in commercial medical (care expenditures: A framework for decomposing price and utilization*. http://www.bea.gov/papers/pdf/RegionalPriceVariation_7_17_11Final.pdf (accessed July 18, 2013).

Farley, P. J. 1985. Who are the underinsured? *Milbank Memorial Fund Quarterly. Health and Society* 476-503.

Farquhar, M. 2008. AHRQ quality indicators. Edited by R. Hughes, Patient safety and quality: An evidence-based handbook for nurses. Rockville, MD: Agency for Healthcare Research and Quality.

Finkelstein, A., S. Taubman, B. Wright, M. Bernstein, J. Gruber, J. P. Newhouse, H. Allen, K. Baicker, and the Oregon Health Study Group. 2012. The Oregon health insurance experiment: Evidence from the first year. *The Quarterly Journal of Economics* 127:1057-1106.

Fiscella, K., P. Franks, M. R. Gold, and C. M. Clancy. 2000. Inequality in quality. *Journal of the American Medical Association* 283(19):2579-2584.

Fisher, E. S., and J. E. Wennberg. 2003. Health care quality, geographic variations, and the challenge of supply-sensitive care. *Perspectives in Biology and Medicine* 46(1):69-79.

Fisher, E. S., J. E. Wennberg, T. A. Stukel, and S. M. Sharp. 1994. Hospital readmission rates for cohorts of Medicare beneficiaries in Boston and New Haven. *New England Journal of Medicine* 331(15):989-995.

Fisher, E. S., D. E. Wennberg, T. A. Stukel, D. J. Gottlieb, F. L. Lucas, and E. L. Pinder. 2003a. The implications of regional variations in Medicare spending. Part 1: The content, quality, and accessibility of care. *Annals of Internal Medicine* 138(4):273-287.

———. 2003b. The implications of regional variations in Medicare spending. Part 2: Health outcomes and satisfaction with care. *Annals of Internal Medicine* 138(4):288-298.

Fisher, E. S., J. P. Bynum, and J. S. Skinner. 2009. Slowing the growth of health care costs—Lessons from regional variation. *New England Journal of Medicine* 360(9):849-852.

Fowler, F. J., P. M. Gallagher, D. L. Anthony, K. Larsen, and J. S. Skinner. 2008. Relationship between regional per capita Medicare expenditures and patient perceptions of quality of care. *Journal of the American Medical Association* 299(20):2406-2412.

Franzini, L., O. I. Mikhail, and J. S. Skinner. 2010. McAllen and El Paso revisited: Medicare variations not always reflected in the under-sixty-five population. *Health Affairs* 29(12):2302-2309.

Frick, A. P., S. G. Martin, and M. Shwartz. 1985. Case-mix and cost differences between teaching and nonteaching hospitals. *Medical Care* 283-295.

Fuchs, V. R., M. B. McClellan, and J. Skinner. 2001. *Area differences in utilization of medical care and mortality among U.S. elderly.* NBER Working Paper 8628. Cambridge, MA: National Bureau of Economic Research.

GAO (Government Accountability Office). 2009. *Medicare physician services: Utilization trends indicate sustained beneficiary acess with high and growing levels of service in some areas of the nation.* Washington, DC: Government Printing Office.

Gold, M. 2004. Geographic variation in Medicare per capita spending: Should policy-makers be concerned? In *The synthesis project: New insights from research results.* Princeton, NJ: Robert Wood Johnson Foundation.

Gold, M., G. Jacobson, A. Damico, and T. Neuman. 2013. Medicare Advantage 2013 spotlight: Enrollment market update. *Kaiser Family Foundation* 8448:2.

Goldman, T. R. 2012. Health policy brief: Eliminating fraud and abuse. *Health Affairs*, July 31.

Gottlieb, D. J., W. Zhou, Y. Song, K. G. Andrews, J. S. Skinner, and J. M. Sutherland. 2010. Prices don't drive regional Medicare spending variations. *Health Affairs* 29(3):537-543.

Harvard University. 2012. *Geographic variation in health care spending, utilization, and quality among the privately insured.* Washington, DC: Institute of Medicine.

Hsu, J., J. Huang, V. Fung, M. Price, R. Brand, R. Hui, B. Fireman, W. Dow, J. Bertko, and J. P. Newhouse. 2009. Distributing $800 billion: An early assessment of Medicare Part D risk adjustment. *Health Affairs* 28(1):215-225.

Kane, R. L., W. C. Lin, and L. A. Blewett. 2002. Geographic variation in the use of post-acute care. *Health Services Research* 37(3):667-682.

Katz, P. 2012. Medicare fraud strike force: Past, present, and future. *Fraud and Abuse* 1(1):1-4.

Manning, W. G., E. C. Norton, and A. S. Wilk. 2012. Explaining geographic variation in health care spending, use and quality, and associated methodological challenges. Paper commissioned by the Committee on Variation in Health Care Spending and Promotion of High-Value Care, Institute of Medicine, Washington, DC. http://www.iom.edu/Reports/2013/Variation-in-Health-Care-Spending-Target-Decision-Making-Not-Geography/~/media/Files/Report%20Files/2013/Geographic-Variation2/Commissioned-Papers/Manning_Norton_Wilk.pdf (accessed August 29, 2013).

MedPAC (Medicare Payment Advisory Commission). 2003. Variation and innovation in Medicare. In *Report to the Congress: June 2003.* Washington, DC: MedPAC.

———. 2008. Reforming the delivery system. In *Report to the Congress: June 2008.* Washington, DC: MedPAC.

———. 2009. Measuring regional variation in service use. In *Report to the Congress: December 2009.* Washington, DC: MedPAC.

———. 2011. Regional variation in Medicare service use. In *Report to the Congress: January 2011.* Washington, DC: MedPAC.

———. 2012. *Health care spending and the Medicare program.* Washington, DC: MedPAC.

Newhouse, J., and Insurance Experiment Group. 1993. *Free for all? Lessons from the RAND health insurance experiment, commercial books.* Cambridge, MA: Harvard University Press.

NQF (National Quality Forum). 2009. National Quality Forum approves criteria for evaluating composite measures. http://www.qualityforum.org/Publications/2013/04/Composite_Performance_Measure_Evaluation_Guidance.aspx (accessed December 30, 2011).

OIG (Office of Inspector General). 2012. *CMS and contractor oversight of home health agencies.* Washington, DC: OIG.

OMB (Office of Management and Budget). 2010. 2010 standards for delineating metropolitan and micropolitan statistical areas; notice. *Federal Register* 75(123):37246-37252.

———. 2013. *Revised delineations of metropolitan statistical areas, micropolitan statistical areas, and combined statistical areas, and guidance on uses of the delineations of these areas.* http://www.whitehouse.gov/sites/default/files/omb/bulletins/2013/b13-01.pdf (accessed March 31, 2013).

PHE (Precision Health Economics, LLC). 2013. *Geographic variation in health care spending and the promotion of high-value care.* Washington, DC: Institute of Medicine.

Pine, M., H. S. Jordan, A. Elixhauser, D. E. Fry, D. C. Hoaglin, B. Jones, R. Meimban, D. Warner, and J. Gonzales. 2007. Enhancement of claims data to improve risk adjustment of hospital mortality. *Journal of the American Medical Association* 297(1):71-76.

Radley, D. 2012. Geographic variation in access to care—The relationship with quality. *New England Journal of Medicine* 367(1):3-6.

Reschovsky, J. D., J. Hadley, C. B. Saiontz-Martinez, and E. R. Boukus. 2011. Following the money: Factors associated with the cost of treating high-cost Medicare beneficiaries. *Health Services Research* 46(4):997-1021.

Sirovich, B. E., D. J. Gottlieb, H. G. Welch, and E. S. Fisher. 2005. Variation in the tendency of primary care physicians to intervene. *Archives of Internal Medicine* 165(19):2252-2256.

Sirovich, B., P. M. Gallagher, D. E. Wennberg, and E. S. Fisher. 2008. Discretionary decision making by primary care physicians and the cost of U.S. health care. *Health Affairs* 27(3):813-823.

Song, Y., J. Skinner, J. Bynum, J. Sutherland, J. E. Wennberg, and E. S. Fisher. 2010. Regional variations in diagnostic practices. *New England Journal of Medicine* 363(1):45-53.

Steinwald, A. B. 2003. *Specialty hospitals: Information on national market share, physician ownership, and patients served.* Letter to the Honorable Bill Thomas, Chairman, Committee on Ways and Means, House of Representatives and the Honorable Jerry Kleczka, House of Representatives. April 18, 2003.

Sutherland, J. M., E. S. Fisher, and J. S. Skinner. 2009. Getting past denial—The high cost of health care in the United States. *New England Journal of Medicine* 361(13):1227-1230.

The Lewin Group. 2013. Geographic variation in health care spending and promotion of high-value care. Washington, DC: Institute of Medicine.

University of Pittsburgh. 2013. *Geographic variation in health care spending and promotion of high-value health care Medicare Part D.* Washington, DC: Institute of Medicine.

Welch, W. P., M. E. Miller, H. G. Welch, E. S. Fisher, and J. E. Wennberg. 1993. Geographic variation in expenditures for physicians' services in the United States. *New England Journal of Medicine* 328(9):621-627.

Wennberg, J. E., and M. M. Cooper. 1998. The surgical treatment of common diseases. In *Dartmouth Atlas of Health Care 1998*. Chicago, IL: American Hospital Publishing. Pp. 108-111.

———. 1999. *The quality of medical care in the United States: A report on the Medicare program. The Dartmouth Atlas of Health Care 1999*. Hanover, NH and Chicago, IL: Dartmouth Medical School and American Hospital Association.

Wennberg, J. E., E. S. Fisher, and J. S. Skinner. 2002. Geography and the debate over Medicare reform. *Health Affairs* Supplemental Web Exclusives W96-W114.

Wennberg, J. E., E. S. Fisher, T. A. Stukel, J. S. Skinner, S. M. Sharp, and K. K. Bronner. 2004. Use of hospitals, physician visits, and hospice care during last six months of life among cohorts loyal to highly respected hospitals in the United States. *British Medical Journal* 328(7440):607.

Wennberg, J. E., S. Brownlee, E. S. Fisher, J. S. Skinner, and J. N. Weinstein. 2008. *An agenda for change: Improving quality and curbing health care spending: Opportunities for the Congress and the Obama administration*. Hanover, NH: Dartmouth Institute for Health Policy and Clinical Practice.

Yuan, Z., G. S. Cooper, D. Einstadter, R. D. Cebul, and A. A. Rimm. 2000. The association between hospital type and mortality and length of stay: A study of 16.9 million hospitalized Medicare beneficiaries. *Medical Care* 38(2):231.

Zuckerman, S., T. Waidmann, R. Berenson, and J. Hadley. 2010. Clarifying sources of geographic differences in Medicare spending. *New England Journal of Medicine* 363(1): 54-62.

Zuckerman, S., T. A. Waidmann, and E. Lawton. 2011. Undocumented immigrants, left out of health reform, likely to continue to grow as share of the uninsured. *Health Affairs* 30(10):1997-2004.

3

Indexing Value in Medicare: The Role of Geographic Area Performance

A n important part of the committee's statement of task focuses on "whether Medicare payment systems should be modified to provide incentives for high-value, high-quality, evidence-based, patient-centered care through adoption of a value index (based on measures of quality and cost) that would adjust payments on a geographic area basis." As described in Chapter 1, the committee defined health care value as the equivalent of net benefit: the amount by which overall health benefit and/ or well-being produced by care exceeds (or falls short of) the costs of producing it. Here "health benefit and/or well-being" and "costs" are assessed as health outcomes and Medicare and other payer spending for goods and services, respectively. To decide whether to recommend Medicare adjustment of provider and hospital payments based on this definition of value, the committee had to define the scope and evaluate the conceptual and empirical dimensions of a geographically based value index.

DEFINING A GEOGRAPHICALLY BASED VALUE INDEX

Value indexes can take specific forms and serve many purposes. In general, a value index is a relative measure of value—for example, a measure of improvement in patient-centered, clinical health outcomes per unit of resources used in one area relative to the national average. In health care, indexes can be used to adjust hospital or provider reimbursement rates based on measures of relative performance. For example, the Centers for Medicare & Medicaid Services' (CMS's) hospital value-based purchasing program and physician payment modifier (authorized under Sections

3001 and 3007 of the Patient Protection and Affordable Care Act [ACA], respectively) adjust hospital and provider payments according to observed hospital and individual provider performance compared with national averages (CMS, 2013a,b).

This chapter focuses primarily on a geographically based value index. Section 1159 of the Affordable Health Care for America Act (H.R. 3962), on which the committee's charge is based, asked the Institute of Medicine (IOM) to consider different value indexes, including a value index that would adjust provider payments based on regional composite measures of quality and cost. Such an index would be designed to encourage high-value care by tying provider reimbursements to the indexed performance of an area.

In earlier legislation, lawmakers in the U.S. House of Representatives and U.S. Senate introduced separate bills (H.R. 2844 and S. 1249, respectively), both entitled the Medicare Payment Improvement Act of 2009. It proposed that a geographically based value index replace the physician work component of the geographic practice cost indexes, which help standardize differences in resource costs (physician work, practice expenses, and malpractice insurance) across geographic areas (CMS, 2010).[1] The geographically based value index, as a relative value ratio, would adjust a portion of provider reimbursements under the Medicare Physician Fee Schedule according to a region's average Medicare Part A and B spending and health care quality for the Medicare population. The bills' sponsors hoped that, by "linking rewards to the outcomes for an entire payment area," providers within a given area would coordinate care, thereby improving health care quality and reducing inefficiencies.[2]

With this historical context in mind, the committee limited its evaluation of a geographically based value index to a relative ratio that would use area-level composite measures of clinical health outcomes and cost to adjust individual hospital and provider payments under Medicare Parts A, B, and D (a *geographic value index*).

CONCEPTUAL ASSESSMENT OF A GEOGRAPHIC VALUE INDEX

The U.S. health care "system" is fragmented at the national, state, community, and practice levels. Rather than networks of interrelated components, it comprises a wide range of smaller health care systems and solo

---

[1]As described in Chapter 1, the IOM produced the report *Geographic Adjustment in Medicare Payment—Phase 1: Improving Accuracy*, which provides recommendations for improving the accuracy of Medicare's current geographic adjustment factors. Detailed descriptions of the geographic practice cost indexes and the hospital wage index are included in that report.

[2]*Health Care Reform*, CR S6491, 111th Cong., Congressional Record 155, no. 87, daily ed. (June 11, 2009).

practitioners operating independently. These systems span diverse populations, providers, and geographic areas, increasing the complexity of the overarching health care system.

Within the U.S. health care system, health care decision making generally occurs at the level of the individual practitioner or organization, such as a hospital or physician group (IOM, 2001, 2010), not at the geographic region level.[3] Payments that target these actors are more likely than those targeting geographic regions to trigger behavioral change because providers will be accountable for the value of health care services delivered (McKethan et al., 2009). Whether a geographic value index is an appropriate policy depends on whether payment modifications pursuant to the payment model effectively shift provider behavior toward greater efficiency (i.e., using fewer resources) without substantially diminishing health care outcomes.

A geographic value index does not target an appropriate level of clinical decision making to trigger behavioral change at the patient-provider level. In fact, a geographic value index is not designed to target any level of actual decision making. Rather, it treats all providers in a geographic area alike, assuming that area-level payment modifications will incentivize the various decision makers within an area to coordinate care and improve efficiencies across the area. However, two practical considerations suggest otherwise.

First, collaboration among competing providers, absent clinical and financial integration, may raise antitrust issues (Kass and Linehan, 2012). Second, payment modifications targeting large areas do not always link individual physician behaviors to spending increases or decreases. Consequently, a physician (or physician group practice) that reduces volume sees not a proportional increase in payment but reduced income (MedPAC, 2007). For example, the sustainable growth rate (SGR) system, which is designed to decrease Medicare Part B spending each year automatically if Medicare expenditures exceed Medicare spending targets in the previous year (and vice versa), has not incentivized providers to constrain spending growth. Rather, overall spending has increased annually since 2003 (Hahn and Mulvey, 2011).[4] Moreover, Medicare's current fee-for-service reimbursement structure allows providers to maintain reimbursement levels despite cuts to individual-service payments by increasing the volume of services provided.

Although setting provider payments by region, as under a geographic

---

[3]Public health measures, such as educational programs, may be directed at the geographic region level. However, such interventions typically are not covered under Medicare and are the domain of public health agencies, such as the Centers for Disease Control and Prevention and state and county health departments (Salinsky, 2010).

[4]The SGR system is an imperfect example because Congress has never allowed payment decreases to take effect when Medicare's actual total expenditures have exceeded targets.

value index, would be more targeted than the current SGR system, it raises similar concerns about altering provider behavior. Regions large enough to have year-to-year stability in spending (e.g., hospital referral regions [HRRs], metropolitan core-based statistical areas [CBSAs]) are in most cases still too large for any individual provider to have enough influence over total expenditures to alter provider behavior patterns (MedPAC, 2007). An exception is when a single delivery system dominates care in an area. In that limited case, payment policies targeting geographically based government units are functionally equivalent to targeting the relevant decision-making unit. However, this scenario does not pertain to the vast majority of the country. Thus, the likelihood that geographically based payments would incentivize all providers in a geographic region to work together to improve value in the region without centralized decision making is low.

In recent years, multiple stakeholders (e.g., payers, providers, employers, local governments) have formed region- or community-based collaboratives focused on improving the value of health care for their populations.[5] In some cases, health care payments may appropriately target these collaboratives. Like accountable care organizations and other integrated organizations, these collaboratives vary in size and organizational structure, and the area they serve may or may not comport with traditional geographic units. Moreover, collaboratives emerge episodically as a result of local initiatives and leadership and are not necessarily tied to central budgets within their communities. Thus, it is unreasonable for long-term payment policies promoting high-value care to use geographic areas as a shortcut for distributing financial resources to health care decision makers within these collaboratives.

Conclusion 3.1. A geographically based value index is unlikely to promote more efficient behaviors among individual providers and thus is unlikely to improve the overall value of health care.

EMPIRICAL ASSESSMENT OF A GEOGRAPHIC VALUE INDEX

A geographic value index for Medicare would have to generate hospital and provider payments perceived as fair. Proponents of a geographic value index argue that paying more (per unit of service or in total) to providers in areas that are better stewards of health care resources and less to providers in regions that are poor stewards is fair policy. Given the fragmented

---

[5]These collaboratives may implement a range of initiatives, including but not limited to improvement in data collection and dissemination, efficient promotion of health service delivery, and provision of financial incentives for high-value care (Alliance for Health Reform, 2013).

structure of health care delivery within the United States, however, area-level payments are fair only under certain conditions. First, all hospitals and providers within an area must be equally deserving of reward (or penalty), implying they behave similarly. Second, assuming that all providers behave similarly, performance levels in high-value areas must be achievable in low-value areas through elimination of inefficiencies. In other words, differences in measured value between low- and high-spending areas cannot include differences stemming from underlying health status and other acceptable sources of variation. As described fully in Chapter 2, the committee commissioned original analyses to test these premises empirically. Relevant results are discussed below.

Variation in Health Care Spending by Unit of Analysis

To determine whether provider organizations within an identified area behave similarly, the committee examined patterns of health care spending across subregions, service types, and clinical condition categories, as well as condition-specific quality measures across HRRs. As noted above, if providers do not behave similarly, a fairness problem arises whereby low-value providers are rewarded simply by virtue of practicing in areas that are on average high-value (the reverse is also true). Starting with HRRs, the committee examined the amount of variation within progressively smaller units of analysis (hospital services area [HSA], hospital, practice, and individual provider levels).

Spending Variation at the Hospital Service Area Level Within Hospital Referral Regions

The committee investigated the extent and range of variation in spending in subregions within HRRs to test whether the HRR is an appropriate geographic unit upon which to base provider payment. HSAs are nested within HRRs, with an average of 11 per HRR, although there is considerable variability (a range of 1 to 76 HSAs per HRR).[6] As one measure of variability within an HRR, the committee examined the ratio of the highest-spending to the lowest-spending HSA within each HRR for HRRs that contain at least three HSAs. At the median (50th percentile) of these ratios, the highest-spending HSA spends 24 percent more than the lowest-spending HSA in the same HRR (Acumen, LLC, 2013, p. 41). In the 76 HRRs with the highest ratios (those above the 75th percentile), the highest-spending

---

[6]Personal communication, Jonathan S. Skinner, Ph.D., Dartmouth Institute for Health Policy and Clinical Practice, Geisel School of Medicine, February 12, 2013.

HSA within each HRR spends at least 36 percent more than the lowest-spending HSA within that HRR.

An analogous assessment decomposed the variance across all HSAs as the sum of variation among HSAs within an HRR and among HRRs. In analyses for the committee, University of Pittsburgh investigators found that about 59 percent of the variation in adjusted HSA Medicare drug spending is within HRRs, compared with 41 percent among HRRs (University of Pittsburgh, 2013, p. 13). Looking at adjusted drug spending, for example, Manhattan (New York) is one of the highest-spending HRRs, while Albuquerque (New Mexico) is one of the lowest-spending, yet the lowest-spending HSA in Manhattan spends less than 25 percent of what is spent by the HSAs within Albuquerque. In addition to heterogeneity in spending within HRRs, there is substantial heterogeneity in utilization patterns.

To illustrate local variation in drug spending and utilization, Pittsburgh investigators calculated that about half of the HSAs located within the borders of HRRs in the highest-drug-spending HRR quintile are not in the highest-drug-spending quintile of HSAs, and approximately half of the HSAs in the lowest-drug-spending quintile of HRRs are not in the lowest-drug-spending quintile of HSAs. Figures 3-1 and 3-2 illustrate this quintile analysis for adjusted drug spending for HRRs and HSAs. The light pink and light blue shaded areas lying outside the heavy lines are, respectively, high- and low-drug-spending HSAs that are not in high- or low-drug-spending HRRs. Conversely, the nonshaded areas within the heavy lines are, respectively, not high- and not low-drug-spending HSAs that lie within high- and low-drug-spending HRRs. In sum, these maps show remarkable misalignment of high- and low-drug-spending HSAs and HRRs.

To quantify further the magnitude of variation occurring at geographic levels smaller than HRRs, Precision Health Economics, LLC (PHE) conducted regression analyses to identify the proportion of HRR-level variation in mean spending and utilization that is attributable to HSAs. As Table 3-1 demonstrates, 45 percent of all HRR-level variation in total Medicare spending occurs among HSAs within HRRs. Overall, PHE found that approximately 40 to 70 percent of variation in spending and utilization remained after controlling for HRR characteristics. Collectively, these findings demonstrate considerable variation in spending and utilization that can be explained not by HRR-level factors but by factors at the smaller, HSA geographic level or even below that level—within HSAs.

Spending Variation at the Hospital Level Within Hospital Referral Regions

Hospitals within the same HRR vary substantially in their resource use, as can be seen from the committee's analysis of Dartmouth data on

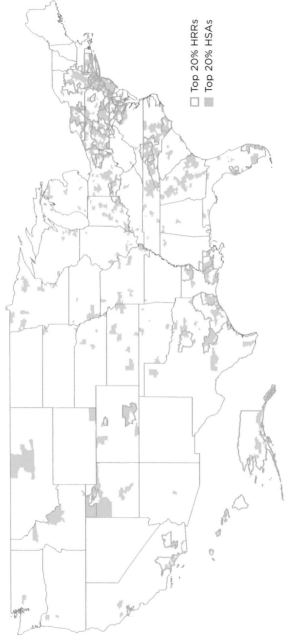

FIGURE 3-1 Top 20 percent of hospital referral regions (HRRs) and hospital service areas (HSAs) in drug spending.

SOURCE: University of Pittsburgh, 2013.

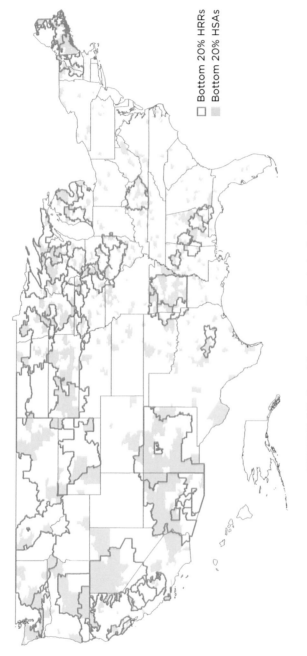

FIGURE 3-2 Bottom 20 percent of hospital referral regions (HRRs) and hospital service areas (HSAs) in drug spending.

SOURCE: University of Pittsburgh, 2013.

Bottom 20% HRRs
Bottom 20% HSAs

TABLE 3-1

Hospital Referral Region Variation in Selected[a] Components of Medicare Spending Attributable to Hospital Services Areas (HSAs)

Spending Component	Proportion of Variation Due to HSAs
Total Spending	0.45
Input-Price-Adjusted Spending	0.41
Inpatient Admissions	0.62
Outpatient Visits	0.52
Prescription Fills	0.56
Emergency Department Visit Days	0.70
Imaging Encounters	0.53

NOTE: Input-price-adjusted spending controls for age, age-sex interaction, partial-year enrollment, year, and health status. Findings are based on a random effects model; results are similar with a fixed-effects model.

[a] The committee was limited in the number of utilization measures it could investigate across Medicare and commercial databases due to time and budget constraints. Hence, post acute care was not included in the committee's main analysis. PHE's analyses reflected those limitations.

SOURCE: Developed by the committee based on data from Precision Health Economics Medicare analysis.

variation in hospital spending for cohorts of patients treated for three major conditions—stroke, hip fracture, and heart attack.[7] Variation among hospitals exists in both lower- and higher-spending HRRs, meaning there are high-spending hospitals in low-spending regions and low-spending hospitals in high-spending regions. Figures 3-3, 3-4, and 3-5, respectively, display observed variation in Medicare spending at the hospital level within each HRR for the above three clinical conditions, after adjustment for input price and health status. The higher the point in the figure, the greater is the variation among hospitals in the HRR. For example, referencing the right-most point in Figure 3-3, in the HRR that spends approximately $45,000 per stroke patient, the difference between spending for hospitals in the 75th and 25th percentiles is around 17 percent of the median value. Differences between hospitals at more extreme points, such as the 90th and 10th percentiles, would, of course, be even larger. In short, Figures 3-3 through 3-5 demonstrate that hospitals within HRRs do not tend to be uniformly high- or low-cost.

---

[7]This analysis was limited to HRRs with four or more hospitals with data on spending for a given condition.

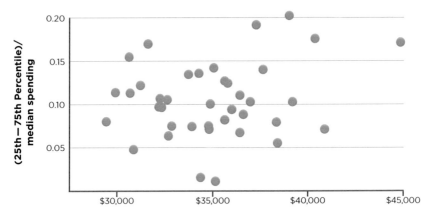

Average spending in HRR for stroke patient

FIGURE 3-3 Variation in price- and risk-adjusted Medicare spending for stroke in a hospital referral region.

SOURCE: Committee analysis of unpublished Dartmouth data (personal communication, Jonathan S. Skinner, Ph.D., Dartmouth Institute for Health Policy and Clinical Practice, Geisel School of Medicine, February 6, 2013).

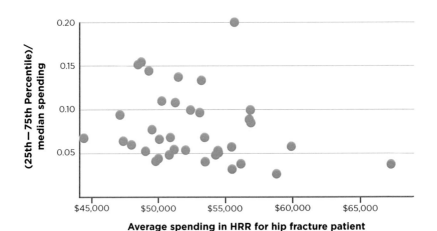

Average spending in HRR for hip fracture patient

FIGURE 3-4 Variation in price- and risk-adjusted Medicare spending for hip fracture in a hospital referral region.

SOURCE: Committee analysis of unpublished Dartmouth data (personal communication, Jonathan S. Skinner, Ph.D., Dartmouth Institute for Health Policy and Clinical Practice, Geisel School of Medicine, February 6, 2013).

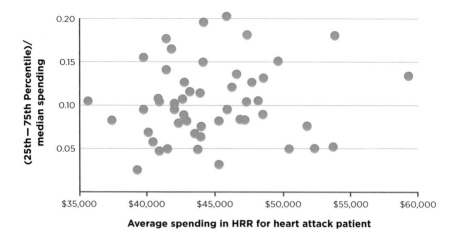

FIGURE 3-5 Variation in price- and risk-adjusted Medicare spending for heart attack in a hospital referral region.

SOURCE: Committee analysis of unpublished Dartmouth data (personal communication, Jonathan S. Skinner, Ph.D., Dartmouth Institute for Health Policy and Clinical Practice, Geisel School of Medicine, February 6, 2013).

Spending Variation Within Provider Practices

Variation also is found among physicians within the same specialty (e.g., cardiology) (Cherkin et al., 1994; Lucas et al., 2010; MedPAC, 2009). The committee could not examine variation below the hospital level (i.e., at the provider level) in its analyses of Medicare data because of restrictions included in data use agreements. Fortunately, commercial insurance data were available. For more than two dozen clinical conditions, Blue Cross Blue Shield of Massachusetts (BCBSMA) regularly examines variation in practice patterns among Massachusetts physicians within particular specialties, comparing physicians with peers in the same practice as well as all comparable specialists across the state. BCBSMA applies episode treatment groups to establish patient populations with defined clinical conditions and then identifies one or two salient differences among physicians in their treatment of those patients. For example, one measure is the tendency of primary care physicians to refer patients with a new episode of knee pain to an orthopedic surgeon. Another is the rate at which cardiologists prescribe angiotensin-converting enzyme (ACE) inhibitors versus more expensive, branded angiotensin receptor blockers for patients with simple hypertension. For each condition, these data indicate that variation among specialists who work in the same group practice is as great as that among

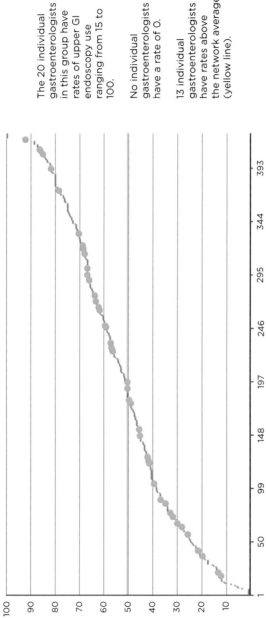

The 20 individual gastroenterologists in this group have rates of upper GI endoscopy use ranging from 15 to 100.

No individual gastroenterologists have a rate of O.

13 individual gastroenterologists have rates above the network average (yellow line).

Individual Gastroenterologists (N=403)

Rate of Upper GI Endoscopy Use per 100 Episodes

FIGURE 3-6 Use of upper gastrointestinal (GI) endoscopy among gastroenterologists treating gastroesophageal reflux disease.

NOTE: Inflammation of the esophagus, without surgery, Group X, 2009. Rate = episodes with upper GI endoscopy/total episode treatment groups.

SOURCE: Personal communication, Dana Gelb Safran, Blue Cross Blue Shield of Massachusetts, July 17, 2011.

specialists across the entire state.[8] For example, Figure 3-6 shows almost as much variation in the use of upper gastrointestinal (GI) endoscopy for patients with gastroesophageal reflux disorder seen by a gastroenterologist (a major driver of spending in that specialty) among 20 physicians within a single practice (denoted by the yellow triangles) as exists for all gastroen- terologists in the state (denoted by the blue dots).[9]

Spending Variation at the Individual Provider Level Across Clinical Conditions

Even individual physician performance varies across different measures of performance. A study by Partners HealthCare of six primary care physi- cians (PCPs) within the same practice group found that individual levels of utilization and quality varied across nine distinct measures associated with diabetes, cholesterol, and hypertension control; ordering of radiology tests and generic prescriptions; and rates of admissions and emergency depart- ment visits (Partners HealthCare, 2012). No single physician was high or low across all measures; instead, each was above average for some and be- low average for others. Similar analyses have been generated for more than 1,100 PCPs and many specialty groups within the Partners Health System. These data demonstrate the difficulty of classifying individual physicians as high- or low-value providers using composite measures. The committee was not provided with standard errors for these analyses, and some of the variation observed is random. Nonetheless, this variation at the physician level suggests that variation among providers within HSAs may be substan- tial, so the foregoing estimates of variation within HRRs attributable to variation among HSAs are a lower bound on variation among all provid- ers within an HRR. In short, it is highly unlikely that all physicians within an HSA practice similarly. As a result, area-level performance calculations would likely mischaracterize the actual value of services delivered by many providers and hospitals, resulting in unfair payments.

Conclusion 3.2. Substantial variation in spending and utilization re- mains as units of analysis get progressively smaller.

---

[8]Personal communication, Dana Gelb Safran, Senior Vice President, Blue Cross Blue Shield of Massachusetts, July 17, 2011.

[9]It should be noted that the patients are likely somewhat heterogeneous, so that some of this variation is attributable to differences in the nature of patients seen by each physician rather than the physician's style of practice. Nonetheless, the variation is, in all likelihood, substantially larger than what patient-level factors could explain when averaged across all patients seen by a physician.

Consistency of Health Care Quality Within an Area

The delivery of health care has become increasingly specialized. Although claims-based quality measures are sparse in some specialized clinical areas, they are plentiful and robust in others (CMS, 2011). Because a geographic value index calculates a composite quality score for a region, many providers in an area will be evaluated on measures not applicable to their practice. Therefore, for a single uniform geographic value index to generate fair reimbursement rates, data would at a minimum have to indicate that performance across a wide range of quality measures was relatively consistent within an area.

Testing this notion, the committee drew on a small sample of the large universe of quality measures, estimating pairwise correlations between 18 condition-specific Medicare quality indicators (Acumen, LLC, 2013, p. 129). Correlations ranged from −0.38 (between diabetes retinal screening and cholecystectomy measures) to 0.67 (between chronic obstructive pulmonary disease [COPD] and congestive heart failure [CHF] admissions). Bivariate correlations showed that approximately 38 percent of quality measures are negatively correlated with each other, 40 percent have correlation coefficients between 0 and 0.19, and only one-fifth have correlation coefficients above 0.20. In short, areas with high scores on some quality measures do not necessarily have high scores on others, particularly if the measures relate to conditions treated by different types of specialists.

To explore the nature of relationships among quality indicators, Harvard examined 31 individual measures: 12 process measures,[10] readmissions within 30 days of discharge (based on Healthcare Effectiveness Data and Information Set [HEDIS] specifications), 12 prevention quality indicators (PQIs) measuring potentially avoidable hospitalizations,[11] and seven patient safety indicators (PSIs) (Harvard University, 2012, pp. 48, 52).[12] HRR-level pairwise correlations between the 10 process measures varied from −0.18 (radiation therapy following breast-conserving therapy and appropriate treatment for low back pain) to 0.52 (antidepressant treatment and treatment with beta blockers following an acute myocardial infarction), but the correlations for most were less than 0.20. The 12 preventable admission rates were highly correlated with each other. Patient safety indicators were not highly correlated (all correlations were less than 0.20).

---

[10]Chosen from the National Committee for Quality Assurance's (NCQA's) 2011 Healthcare Effectiveness Data and Information Set (HEDIS) or recommended by the relevant specialty society.

[11]These measures were developed by the Agency for Healthcare Research and Quality (AHRQ) and were designed to measure the quality of ambulatory care.

[12]These measures were also developed by AHRQ and were designed to measure adverse events associated with medical errors.

And correlations across measure types (for example, process measures with preventable hospitalizations) were generally low, with a few exceptions (Harvard University, 2013).

Collectively, these findings suggest that an area in which providers deliver high-value treatment for one condition may well contain providers who deliver low-value treatment for other conditions. This finding again demonstrates that provider performance within an area is not homogeneous.

Consistency of Health Care Spending and Utilization Within an Area

Spending and utilization measures across conditions are more highly correlated within an HRR than are the quality measures just described (see Tables 3-2 and 3-3). Nonetheless, an HRR that uses many services to treat a given condition (e.g., prostate cancer) does not necessarily use many services to treat another (e.g., low back pain). In that example, the correlation across HRRs for Medicare beneficiaries is 0.485 and for the commercial population is 0.43.

Conclusion 3.3. Quality across conditions and treatments varies widely within HRRs; spending and utilization across conditions are moderately correlated within HRRs.

"Acceptable" and "Unacceptable" Sources of Geographic Variation

Some proponents of a geographic value index contend that area-level payments may be appropriate even if provider behavior varies within an area, reasoning that after controlling for acceptable sources of variation, any remaining variation represents inefficiencies correctable through area-level payment incentives. To evaluate this assertion, the committee commissioned analyses (see Chapter 2) to identify potential sources of variation and quantify their possible influences.[13] It is important to underscore again here that characterizing this unexplained variation as "acceptable" or "unacceptable" is impossible, as associated sources cannot be observed within the available data. As established by the detailed results and related discussion in Chapter 2, however, the robustness of this body of findings points to important residual variation in health care spending and utilization, indicative of inefficiencies not necessarily remediable at the geographic level.

---

[13]Note that unacceptable variation can arise from both overuse and underuse.

TABLE 3-2
Pearson Correlation Coefficients for Medicare Beneficiary Utilization (Risk-Adjusted Per-Member-Per-Month Cost) Across Cohorts

	Lower Back Pain	Cataracts	Congestive Heart Failure	Breast Cancer	Prostate Cancer	Cholecystectomy
Lower Back Pain	1.00					
Cataracts	0.477	1.00				
Congestive Heart Failure	0.907	0.483	1.00			
Breast Cancer	0.574	0.311	0.583	1.00		
Prostate Cancer	0.485	0.230	0.502	0.524	1.00	
Cholecystectomy	0.593	0.353	0.624	0.406	0.406	1.00

SOURCE: Acumen, LLC, 2013.

TABLE 3-3
Pearson Correlation Coefficients for Input-Price-Adjusted Spending Across Cohorts in the Harvard MarketScan Commercial Population

	Lower Back Pain	Cataracts	Congestive Heart Failure	Breast Cancer	Prostate Cancer	Cholecystectomy
Lower Back Pain	1.00					
Cataracts	0.35	1.00				
Congestive Heart Failure	0.52	0.36	1.00			
Breast Cancer	0.49	0.52	0.37	1.00		
Prostate Cancer	0.43	0.33	0.39	0.49	1.00	
Cholecystectomy	0.40	0.36	0.39	0.42	0.36	1.00

SOURCE: Harvard University, 2012.

Relationships Between Spending or Utilization and Quality

Use of a geographic value index would require that area-level performance be observable in reliable relationships between health care resource use and health care quality. Absent such reliable relationships, geographically based value adjustment would have, on balance, no predictable effect on overall quality. Thus, assuming that composite measures of health care spending and health outcomes are used to measure value, the case for an area-wide payment adjuster is stronger if a payment change has consistent effects on the quality measures making up the composites.

The committee's commissioned analyses did not reveal a consistent relationship between condition-specific utilization and area-wide condition-specific quality measures in the Medicare population. The measures are scaled such that a positive correlation indicates that higher condition-specific utilization is associated with higher-quality care. Positive correlations between quality and utilization varied from 0.005 for radiation therapy for breast cancer to 0.085 for disease-modifying antirheumatic drugs dispensed for arthritis (0.085). Negative correlations between quality and utilization varied from −0.012 for antiplatelet prescription over 12 months for coronary heart disease (CHD) to −0.483 for bronchodilator prescription 30 days following an acute COPD event (Acumen, LLC, 2013, pp. 104-111, 131).

In the commercial population, Harvard found that positive correlations between quality measures and spending varied from 0.02 for the preventable acute admissions composite to 0.30 for antibiotics following pneumonia diagnosis (Harvard University, 2012, pp. 19-21, 58). Negative correlations between quality and spending ranged from −0.07 for readmissions and the preventable admissions composite to −0.13 for the preventable chronic admissions composite. Spending, however, can be disaggregated into price and quantity components. Holding input price constant and focusing on variation in the quantity of services, positive correlations between utilization and quality ranged from 0.06 for breast cancer screening mammography to 0.09 for readmissions. Negative correlations between utilization and quality varied from −0.06 for antibiotics following pneumonia diagnosis to −0.57 for imaging following complaint of low back pain (Harvard University, 2012, pp. 18-23, 58).

Although the committee believes several of these correlations are subject to measurement error because of small samples, there is no affirmative evidence of a consistent relationship between spending and quality. Few of the correlations differ substantially from zero.[14]

---

[14]This is so even though mechanical relationships between quality measures and utilization cause some correlations to be artificially strong. For example, the outcome for the COPD admissions quality measure is an inpatient admission. As the rate of COPD admissions increases in a region, indicating a lower quality of COPD care, utilization, by definition, necessarily increases.

In sum, acknowledging the limitations and challenges to interpretation of the quality analyses, overall the committee found no evidence of reliable associations between disease- or condition-specific measures of utilization and disease- or condition-specific measures of quality. As a result, a geographic value index employing these measures could affect some health outcomes negatively and others positively.

Findings from the committee's commissioned empirical analyses are consistent with those of a recent systematic review demonstrating an inconsistent relationship between health care quality and cost (Hussey et al., 2013). Of 61 studies selected for review, 21 (34 percent) found a positive or mostly positive association, 18 (30 percent) found a negative or mostly negative association, and 22 (36 percent) found an inconsistent or no association between health care quality and cost. Further, the authors of the review concluded that the magnitude of the cost-quality association was generally low or moderate from the perspective of clinical significance.

Conclusion 3.4. HRR-level quality is not consistently related to spending or utilization in Medicare or the commercial sector.

It is important to note that this particular conclusion is limited to area-level, composite measures of value derived from administrative claims data and should not be interpreted as condemning initiatives to improve health care value. Nor does it imply that particular providers in low- or high-cost areas currently are being compensated appropriately.

RECOMMENDATION 2: Congress should not adopt a geographically based value index for Medicare. Because geographic units are not where most health care decisions are made, a geographic value index would be a poorly targeted mechanism for encouraging value improvement. Adjusting payments geographically, based on any aggregate or composite measure of spending or quality, would unfairly reward low-value providers in high-value regions and punish high-value providers in low-value regions.

REFERENCES

Acumen, LLC. 2013. *Geographic variation in spending, utilization and quality: Medicare and Medicaid beneficiaries.* Washington, DC: Institue of Medicine.
Alliance for Health Reform. 2013. *Select community quality initiatives map.* http://allhealth. org/community-initiatives.asp (accessed February 19, 2013).
Cherkin, D. C., R. A. Deyo, K. Wheeler, and M. A. Ciol. 1994. Physician variation in diagnostic testing for low back pain. Who you see is what you get. *Arthritis & Rheumatism* 37(1):15-22.

CMS (Centers for Medicare & Medicaid Services). 2010. Medicare program: Payment policies under the physician fee schedule and other revisions for Part B for CY 2011. *Federal Register* 75(288):73170-73860.

———. 2011. *Claims-based quality measures.* http://www.cms.gov/Medicare/Medicare-Fee-for-Service-Payment/PhysicianFeedbackProgram/downloads/claims_based_measures_with_descriptions_num_denom_excl.pdf (accessed July 18, 2013)

———. 2013a. *Hospital value-based purchasing.* http://www.cms.gov/Medicare/Quality-Initiatives-Patient-Assessment-Instruments/hospital-value-based-purchasing/index.html?redirect=/hospital-value-based-purchasing (accessed April 4, 2013).

———. 2013b. *Value-based payment modifier.* http://www.cms.gov/Medicare/Medicare-Fee-for-Service-Payment/PhysicianFeedbackProgram/ValueBasedPaymentModifier.html (accessed April 4, 2013).

Hahn, J., and J. Mulvey. 2011. *Medical physician payment updates and the sustainable growth rate (SGR) system.* Washington, DC: Congressional Research Service.

Harvard University. 2012. *Geographic variation in health care spending, utilization, and quality among the privately insured.* Washington, DC: Institute of Medicine.

———. 2013. *Harvard HRR-level quality measures correlations.* Washington, DC: Institute of Medicine.

Hussey, P. S., S. Wertheimer, and A. Mehrotra. 2013. The association between health care quality and cost: A systematic review. *Annals of Internal Medicine* 158(1):27-34.

IOM (Institute of Medicine). 2001. *Crossing the quality chasm: A new health system for the 21st century.* Washington, DC: National Academy Press.

———. 2010. *Leadership commitments to improve value in health care: Finding common ground: Workshop summary.* Washington, DC: The National Academies Press.

Kass, J. E., and J. S. Linehan. 2012. Fostering healthcare reform through a bifurcated model of fraud and abuse regulation. *Journal of Health & Life Sciences Law* 5(75):79-93.

Lucas, F. L., B. E. Sirovich, P. M. Gallagher, A. E. Siewers, and D. E. Wennberg. 2010. Variation in cardiologists' propensity to test and treat: Is it associated with regional variation in utilization? *Circulation: Cardiovascular Quality and Outcomes* 3(3):253-260.

McKethan, A., M. Shepard, S. L. Kocot, N. Brennan, M. Morrison, N. Nguyen, R. D. Williams, and N. Cafarella. 2009. *Improving quality and value in the U.S. health care system.* Washington, DC: Engelberg Center for Health Reform, Brookings Institution, and Avalere Health, LLC.

MedPAC (Medicare Payment Advisory Commission). 2007. *Assessing alternatives to the sustainable growth rate system.* Washington, DC: MedPAC.

———. 2009. Measuring regional variation in service use. In *Report to the Congress: December 2009.* Washington, DC: MedPAC.

Partners HealthCare. 2012. *Variation within a single group of primary care physicians at Partners Healthcare, Inc.* Boston, MA: Partners HealthCare, Inc.

Salinsky, E. 2010. *Governmental public health: An overview of state and local public health agencies.* Washington, DC: National Health Policy Forum.

University of Pittsburgh. 2013. *Geographic variation in health care spending and promotion of high-value health care Medicare Part D.* Washington, DC: Institute of Medicine.

4

Payment and Organizational Reforms to Improve Value

The delivery of health care involves myriad decisions made by a wide range of decision makers, including solo practitioners, single-specialty group practices, multiple-specialty group practices, hospitals, health care systems, and in some cases community-based multistakeholder collaboratives (Sennett et al., 2011; Share et al., 2011; Shih et al., 2008). As discussed in detail in Chapter 3, the committee's research, analyses, and deliberations led to the conclusion that Congress should relate provider payments to outcomes arising from the actions of specific health care decision makers rather than to average outcomes in geographic areas. Perhaps the most important reason to target policies at decision makers is that incentives would otherwise be misdirected; an area-level payment incentive, for example, might do little to cause an individual physician or hospital to seek efficiency in delivering care.

Misdirected incentives are not the only reason to favor payment policies targeting providers. The committee's research and analyses revealed how variation in spending and quality exists in progressively smaller units, down to the hospital, single-specialty group practice, and even individual physician level, suggesting that opportunities exist for improving value at all levels of health care decision making.[1] Decision makers differ in their abilities to maximize efficiency and improve value (Audet et al., 2005; Goldberg et al., 2013; Landon et al., 1998; Shih et al., 2008; Sterns, 2007). For example, an individual practitioner or small group practice can

---

[1]See the committee's conceptualization of value, given the current state of the art, in Chapter 1, pp 8-9.

take small-scale steps to improve quality and efficiency (e.g., by following evidence-based guidelines or recommending equally efficacious lower-cost treatments to patients) (Wolfson et al., 2009). Group practices, hospitals, health care organizations, and multistakeholder collaboratives, on the other hand, can track and manage patient care across many providers (to different degrees) and may be able to improve value through broader initiatives—for example, through efforts that increase care coordination and target high-risk individuals for disease management programs (Paulus et al., 2008; Shih et al., 2008). As Guterman and colleagues (2009) argue, citing such examples as Geisinger Health System, the North Carolina Community Care model of medical homes, and Medicare's Physician Group Practice Demonstration, when providers are accountable for a broader continuum of health care for their populations, they can increase the value of the care they deliver (Guterman et al., 2009).

Payers can help align the financial goals of these health care decision makers with high-value care. Today in traditional Medicare, the Centers for Medicare & Medicaid Services (CMS) largely pays physicians on a fee-for-service basis and pays hospitals using the diagnosis-related group (DRG) system (a form of bundled payment for inpatient services and diagnoses). Because of the importance of Medicare, many providers find it convenient to contract with private insurers using the same methods (Mayes and Berenson, 2006). Such a payment system does not promote high-value care for several reasons. First, because providers are paid for the number and intensity of services rendered, not for treating patients efficiently and effectively, fee-for-service payment does not reward providers for sharing information or coordinating care plans. In fact, coordination of care in this environment often penalizes health care providers financially, as providing health care more efficiently means reducing the number of services charged for (Enthoven, 2009; McClellan, 2011; MedPAC, 2012a; Miller, 2007) and may result in a loss of competitive position in a local market. Consequently, "there is little systematic coordination of a patient's care among multiple providers and settings" (MedPAC, 2012a, p. 36). Second, since all financial risk in fee-for-service payment is relegated to the payer, providers have no financial incentive (and often have a financial disincentive) to select equally efficacious lower-cost care options (McClellan, 2011). Finally, beneficiary cost sharing in traditional Medicare and for the most part under private insurance is unrelated to the benefit of services. Patients, like physicians, have no financial incentive to select lower-cost treatment options that may be equally efficacious (Partnership for Sustainable Health Care, 2013).

The statement of task for this study asked the committee to recommend payment reforms that would promote the delivery of high-value care, taking into consideration the Patient Protection and Affordable Care Act (ACA)

(P.L. 111-148)[2] and related changes already under way. Medicare payment reform has the potential to promote high-value care by encouraging provider organizations to develop the capacity to manage the continuum of care for their patient populations efficiently. The following sections address in turn (1) the importance of clinical and financial integration to building a high-value health care delivery system, and how payment reforms are designed to promote such integration; (2) why, under the tenets of a learning health care system,[3] it is important for CMS to evaluate and refine new payment models; and (3) strategies for encouraging broader adoption of new payment reforms.

BUILDING A HIGH-VALUE HEALTH CARE SYSTEM THROUGH CLINICAL AND FINANCIAL INTEGRATION

Fragmentation characterizes the organization and delivery of health care services in the United States at the national, state, community, and practice levels (Shih et al., 2008). With no overarching system as a guide, health care services are delivered across an increasing array of distinct and often competing providers and entities, each with different objectives, obligations, and capabilities (Cebul et al., 2008). Providers practicing within the same geographic area, sometimes caring for the same patients, often work independently from and not communicating with one another (Bodenheimer, 2008; Shih et al., 2008).

Increasingly, this fragmented health care delivery system is ill equipped to manage the continuum of health care for an aging population with complex needs. In 2010, 21 million (68.4 percent) and 11 million (36.4 percent) Medicare beneficiaries (in Traditional Medicare Part A and B) had two and four or more chronic conditions, respectively (Lochner and Cox, 2013). Beneficiaries with multiple chronic conditions are the most frequent and intensive users of Medicare services; they see on average as many as three primary care physicians and eight specialists, and typically receive care in seven unique health care facilities (Pham et al., 2007). Understandably, care coordination for these patients is exceedingly difficult, as indicated by a 2009 Robert Wood Johnson Foundation finding that for every 100 Medicare patients treated, coordinating care would require that

---

[2]Patient Protection and Affordable Care Act, Public Law 111-148, 111th Cong., 2nd sess. (March 23, 2010).

[3]A learning health care system is defined as "a health care system that generates and applies the best evidence for the collaborative health care choices of each patient and provider; drives the process of discovery as a natural outgrowth of patient care; and ensures innovation, quality, safety, and value in health care" (Institute of Medicine [IOM] Roundtable on Value & Science-Driven Health Care Charter).

each primary care physician communicate with 99 other physicians in 53 practice locations (Pham, 2009). According to Guterman, "Currently, even when individual services meet high standards of clinical quality, there is often insufficient coordination of care across settings and over time to meet the needs of patients" (Guterman et al., 2011, p. 9).

Fragmentation, particularly in the context of chronic or comorbid conditions, spurs inefficiency through a lack of information sharing, duplicate testing, poor care coordination, and mismanagement of care transitions (American Hospital Association, 2010b; IOM, 2012; Shih et al., 2008; Stremikis et al., 2011). The Institute of Medicine's (IOM's) Committee on the Learning Health Care System in America concluded, "Chronic diseases and comorbid conditions are increasing, exacerbating the clinical, logistical, decision-making, and economic challenges faced by patients and clinicians" (IOM, 2012, p. S5).

What Health Care Systems Can Do

A growing body of evidence supports the corollary to the consequences of fragmentation that clinical and financial integration best positions health care systems to manage the continuum of care for their complex populations efficiently (Casalino et al., 2003; Chuang et al., 2004; Landon, 1998; McWilliams et al., 2013; Moullec et al., 2012; Shih et al., 2008; Sterns, 2007). Clinical integration denotes a minimum level of coordination and alignment of goals among providers (physicians, hospitals, and other practitioners) caring for a population (Burns and Muller, 2008). In clinically integrated environments, providers share clinical data, agree on plans of care, and collaborate to achieve favorable patient-centered outcomes. Hence, at a minimum, they must foster care coordination among individual providers of care, as well as share data and track service use and outcomes to measure progress (Shortell et al., 1994). Financial integration often hastens clinical integration. Financially integrated health care systems have the capability to receive payments and distribute them to individual care providers, which in turn allows health care systems to align financial incentives among providers within organizations (Hastings, 2012). However, financial integration is not a unitary goal; historically, financially integrated health care organizations lacking management, infrastructure, and processes to coordinate care (i.e., clinical integration) generally have not succeeded in substantially lowering costs or improving care quality, and sometimes have completely failed in this regard (Frakt and Mayes, 2012).

Health care systems in which physician groups and hospitals are under the same ownership (integrated at the corporate level) reflect one common organizational model, but clinical and financial integration exists across a large spectrum of relationships among hospitals, practitioners, and other entities (Guterman et al., 2011; Shih et al., 2008). Group model health maintenance or prepaid health organizations represent one well-established form of integration (Gaynor et al., 2001). In recent years, moreover, formerly independent or loosely linked providers have pursued tighter integration (Advocate Health Care, 2013). One example is Fairview Health Services (FHS), an academic medical center in Minneapolis. It embarked on a clinical and financial integration program[4] across all partnering physicians, even though their practices reflect varying relationships with FHS. These relationships include (1) 500 primary care physicians employed by FHS, (2) 700 specialist physicians within the University of Minnesota practice plan, (3) 1,000 primary care and specialty physicians belonging to a physician hospital organization, and (4) 1,500 primary and specialty physicians practicing independently (American Hospital Association, 2010b).

Maintaining a robust health information technology infrastructure is crucial for both clinical and financial integration. Electronic health records (EHRs), data warehousing, and analytics (leveraging data captured in EHRs) are critical for providers to receive timely quality and cost data with which to track their performance, and were considered essential for the successful implementation of bundled payment in the PROMETHEUS experiment[5] (Hussey et al., 2011). An emerging body of studies suggests that provider use of health information technology (HIT) may help improve disease management and care coordination processes and positively impact health outcomes, especially for patients with multiple chronic conditions (Cebul et al., 2011; Herrin et al., 2012; Kern et al., 2012). Further, well-designed EHRs can promote care coordination by increasing providers' access to patient information and support high-quality care by incorporating evidence-based clinical pathways (Mechanic and Zinner, 2012). Providers and hospitals have made significant progress in adopting HIT systems; however, much more remains to be done. As of 2011, just over half of physicians had adopted EHRs (Decker et al., 2012; Jamoom et al., 2012), 75 percent of which met minimum federal standards.[6]

One caveat of note is that clinical and financial integration may in some

---

[4]FHS's quality improvement and cost reduction program has two main components: (1) "care packages" detailing best practices for 12 conditions and procedures (e.g., low back pain, diabetes, prenatal care, knee replacement), and (2) a shift in provider reimbursement away from fee-for-service to a single fee covering the entire package of services (American Hospital Association, 2010a).

[5]PROMETHEUS, an acronym for Provider Payment Reform for Outcomes, Margins, Evidence, Transparency, Hassle Reduction, Excellence, Understandability and Sustainability, is a bundled payment pilot project. Its development and evaluation were sponsored by The Commonwealth Fund and the Robert Wood Johnson Foundation (Hussey et al., 2011).

[6]CMS provides incentives to providers who make "meaningful use" of EHRs. The requirements for meaningful use are available at https://www.cms.gov/Regulations-and-Guidance/Legislation/EHRIncentivePrograms/Meaningful_Use.html.

markets increase provider concentration (a potential violation of antitrust laws), enabling providers in those markets to charge commercial carriers higher prices (RWJF, 2012).[7] Antitrust enforcement often raises a difficult trade-off between production efficiencies and market power, and health care is no exception (RWJF, 2012). Nonetheless, greater value clearly requires greater coordination among providers.

What Payers Can Do

Payers can promote value through payment and organizational reforms that foster the above elements of clinical and financial integration. In fact, many payment reforms included in the ACA and tested in the commercial market (e.g., value-based purchasing [VBP], bundled payment, accountable care organizations [ACOs], patient-centered medical home (PCMH) models, and dual-eligible care integration demonstrations, all discussed later in this chapter) do just that. Early provider reaction has been positive, as reflected in the larger-than-anticipated number of organizations contracting with CMS to join pilot programs (CMS, 2013f; Muhlestein, 2013). However, the U.S. health care delivery system spans a diverse array of provider organizational relationships, which vary in size, level of integration (both clinical and financial), and ability/willingness to assume financial risk (Guterman, 2010). The Commonwealth Foundation developed a graph (see Figure 4-1) depicting the interaction between provider organizational models and alternative payment mechanisms. Because these reforms are relatively new, evidence on their influence on value, particularly in less integrated organizational settings, is limited. Therefore, it would be advisable for CMS to test payment models that are compatible with less as well as more clinically integrated providers to see how reforms impact the value of care in different settings (Guterman and Drake, 2010).

Also critical is for payers, including CMS, to make real-time data on service use and relative performance levels available to provider organizations. To identify opportunities for improving value, providers require ongoing data collection and analysis concerning the effects of value improvement interventions. Where regional collaboratives have constructed multipayer databases, data on Medicare patients have generally been excluded or out of date. According to Miller (2011, p. 14), "In the few communities where Medicare data has been made available, it has typically

---

[7]The increase in commercial payments would raise total health care spending directly. But if Medicare kept its prices at some proportion of commercial prices, say 80 percent, it would also spend more; if it did not do so, Medicare beneficiaries might experience access problems since the gap between commercial and Medicare payments in such markets would be particularly large.

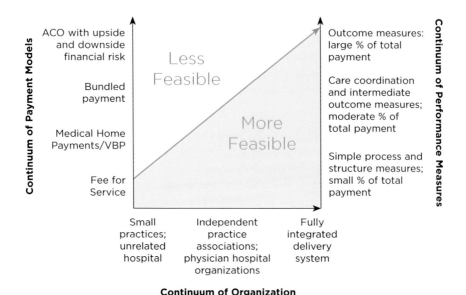

FIGURE 4-1 Organization and payment methods.

NOTE: "Global case" is equivalent to bundled payment (discussed in the text). P4P = pay for performance.

SOURCE: Adapted from The Commonwealth Fund, 2008.

been several years old. Data that are out-of-date are of relatively little value in communities where there are active efforts to improve the quality and cost of care; indeed, using old data can be counterproductive since it may unfairly imply that problems exist when, in reality, they have already been addressed."

What Patients Can Do

Finally, patients are also health care decision makers and can be encouraged through alternative cost-sharing arrangements to share in the savings of higher-value care. In this connection, it is important to acknowledge that "clinical services vary in the value they provide to patients, and that not all patients with a specific clinical condition receive the same level of benefit from a specific intervention" (Fendrick and Chernew, 2006, p. SP10). There is little debate that cost sharing (increasing or decreasing patients' out-of-pocket costs) influences the use of health care services (Fendrick and Chernew, 2006). Introducing value-based cost sharing into a health care system may encourage patients to frequent high-value providers and/ or higher-value care options. However, increasing cost sharing has been shown to decrease the use of both effective and ineffective services; thus, more information is needed on how best to tailor a program to encourage the selection of higher-value care options (IOM, 2012). CMS should therefore consider piloting programs that seek to align patient cost-sharing arrangements with value.

> **RECOMMENDATION 3: To improve value, the Centers for Medicare & Medicaid Services (CMS) should continue to test payment reforms that incentivize the clinical and financial integration of health care delivery systems and thereby encourage their (1) coordination of care among individual providers, (2) real-time sharing of data and tracking of service use and health outcomes, (3) receipt and distribution of provider payments, and (4) assumption of some or all of the risk of managing the care continuum for their populations. Further, CMS should pilot programs that allow beneficiaries to share in the savings due to higher-value care.**

EVALUATING AND REFINING NEW PAYMENT MODELS

Payment reforms can target the full spectrum of health care decision makers, encouraging individual providers in highly fragmented areas to maximize their own efficiencies and coordinate with each other while allowing more organized health care systems and collaboratives to assume additional risk (and potential reward) in managing the health of their patient populations (IOM, 2012; Shih et al., 2008). This can be done directly by paying health care providers that achieve selected quality and efficiency metrics (e.g., VBP) or implement care coordination programs (e.g., PCMHs), or indirectly by shifting some or all financial risk to health care systems (e.g., bundled payment, ACOs, Medicare Advantage plans). Many payment and organizational reforms include both of the above strategies; in the Pioneer program, for example, ACOs must achieve specific quality measures as well as assume some financial risk (CMS, 2012). The following sections briefly offer the rationale for and evidence supporting selected payment reforms in the ACA and illustrate why it is necessary to continue testing and refining new payment models before generalizing them to the broader Medicare population.

Value-Based Purchasing

In Medicare, the program now known as VBP began as pay-for-reporting (paying providers for reporting quality data) and then was called pay-for-performance (paying providers for meeting quality standards). The newer VBP models require providers to meet quality and cost reduction goals (paying for efficiency or value). One benefit of VBP is that it can target any level of health care decision making, including individual practitioners (Folsom et al., 2008).

Pay-for-performance and VBP have been touted as effective interventions for improving health care outcomes, yet evaluation results are mixed. Although a large-scale Medicare hospital demonstration of pay-for-performance showed promise in the first 2 years (Lindenauer et al., 2007), quality improvement, as indicated by reductions in mortality, was not achieved over the full 6-year duration of the program (Jha et al., 2012; Ryan et al., 2012; Werner et al., 2011). Similarly, the United Kingdom's universal pay-for-performance program for primary care physicians, implemented in 2004, showed improved results on all quality measures in the first year, but several measures subsequently leveled off (Campbell et al., 2009; Doran et al., 2011).

More than 40 private-sector pay-for-performance programs operate throughout the United States. One example, Integrated Health Association's (IHA's) California Pay-for-Performance Program, is the largest private physician incentive program in the United States (James, 2012). Rosenthal and colleagues (2005) evaluated how California physician groups participating in the program (intervention group) compared to Pacific Northwest physician groups (control group) on three quality measures (cervical cancer screening, mammography, and hemoglobin A1c testing) (Rosenthal et al., 2005). Although the intervention group improved on all three quality measures over the course of the study, control comparisons showed the intervention group's quality to be higher only for the cervical cancer screening measure. The authors concluded that the study results do not justify the program's price tag of $3.4 million. In a complementary follow-up study, Mullen and colleagues (2008) concluded that overall, the program resulted in a "small and mixed return on investment" (Mullen et al., 2008, p. 26). More specifically, Mullen and colleagues concluded that the size of incentives matters. IHA's program will be transitioning to include value-based cost measures starting in 2014 (Dolan and Yanagihara, 2011).

CMS launched a Medicare hospital-based VBP program in October 2012. Evaluation measures for the program's first year include process measures and patient satisfaction; CMS plans to extend these measures to include health outcomes and costs. Hospitals are eligible for incentives based on overall achievement and improvement relative to previous years. Program funding comes from a 1 percent withhold from regular fee-for-service payments to participating hospitals; this withhold increases each year up to 2 percent in 2017 and beyond. The level of incentive payments depends on hospital performance. CMS estimates that about half of hospitals will see a net increase in payments, but expected changes in payment are small even for best and worst performers (Werner and Dudley, 2012).

Although VBP has not yet been shown to produce substantial improvements in health care value, it does encourage providers and health care organizations to invest in the HIT systems needed to track patient cost and care measures (Folsom et al., 2008). In conjunction with other payment changes, therefore, it may produce value in other ways.

Patient-Centered Medical Homes

The PCMH is a health care delivery model that organizes the care continuum around a practitioner team with the primary care provider at the center, helping patients coordinate care and manage chronic conditions. The PCMH also generally incorporates evidence-based medicine and quality improvement activities (Cassidy, 2010; Jackson et al., 2013). Proponents believe the PCMH will reduce care costs and improve quality. For example, one analysis of 43 primary care clinics participating in the Geisinger ProvenHealth Navigator project between 2006 and 2010 found that increased length of time in the program was significantly associated with lower total cost and with the total cumulative cost savings over the study period of 4.3 to 7.1 percent (Maeng et al., 2012). Group Health Cooperative of Seattle estimates that it generated a return of $1.50 for every $1 invested in its medical home demonstration (Reid, 2010).

The PCMH model has been widely implemented by provider organizations, CMS, and other third-party payers. By 2011, more than 1,500 provider practices nationwide had received medical home recognition from the National Committee for Quality Assurance (NCQA) (NCQA, 2011).[8]

CMS currently is participating in three PCMH initiatives. First, under the Medicare Multi-Payer Advanced Primary Care Demonstration, CMS is joining state reform initiatives involving multiple payers (including Medicaid and private health plans) by paying a monthly care management fee for beneficiaries receiving medical home care. This program, operating in eight

---

[8]NCQA created a self-report evaluation for physician practices, which has become the evaluation tool used to judge most ongoing demonstrations. This tool has three levels and assesses nine standards: access and communication, patient tracking and registries, care management, patient self-management support, electronic prescribing, test tracking, referral tracking, performance reporting and improvement, and advanced electronic communications.

states over a 3-year period, covers more than 1,200 provider practices and nearly 1 million beneficiaries (CMS, 2013g). Second, CMS, partnering with the Health Resources and Services Administration (HRSA), supports the Federally Qualified Health Center (FQHC) Advanced Primary Care Practice Demonstration, which pays a monthly care management fee for each eligible Medicare beneficiary receiving primary care services through 1 of 492 FQHCs meeting NCQA requirements for a medical home. CMS and HRSA also will provide technical assistance (e.g., webinars on quality standards) to help FQHCs achieve quality and cost goals (CMS, 2013e). Finally, the Comprehensive Primary Care Initiative is another multipayer program, in which CMS and participating private insurers give primary care providers bonus payments for improving care coordination (CMS, 2013c).

A small but growing body of research is devoted to evaluating the effects of the PCMH model. A recent review of 19 studies revealed "moderately strong evidence suggest[ing] that the medical home has a small positive effect on patient experiences and small to moderate positive effects on preventive care services" (Jackson et al., 2013, p. 175). According to the authors, however, current evidence is insufficient to determine how the PCMH will influence most clinical and economic outcomes.

Bundled Payment

Under bundled payment, a payer makes a single payment for all services (a bundle) provided during an episode of care. The definition of an episode of care is challenging and fundamental to the implementation of this payment approach (Hussey et al., 2012). Episodes of care range from single acute medical conditions to periods of treatment for chronic disease. Bundled payment targets an entity (e.g., hospital, health care organization or network) capable of receiving payment, which then divides the payment among those providing episode-based care (e.g., the hospital, the laboratory, physicians, post-acute care providers) (CMS, 2013b; Pham et al., 2010). If patients are treated by providers not affiliated with the entity receiving the bundled payment, payers may reimburse those providers on a fee-for-service basis, adjusting each payment to the overarching organization so that total payment to all service providers does not exceed a predefined bundled cost. This process is referred to as "virtual" bundling (American Medical Association, 2012). Bundled payment approaches usually incorporate quality measures, increasing provider payments when quality standards are met.

Proponents note that bundled payment has the potential to decrease health care waste by reducing incentives to provide unnecessary services as part of an episode of care and increasing care coordination (Burton, 2012). More specifically, if bundled payment includes services received from multiple providers, such as physicians, hospitals, and post-acute care providers, incentives are offered to coordinate care (share information), shift care to more efficient providers, and reduce duplicative tests and unnecessary physician visits (Painter, 2013).

As previously stated, CMS's long-standing (since 1983) inpatient DRG payment system is a form of bundled payment in that it bundles facility-only services for a given hospital stay. By no longer paying hospitals per diem, the DRG system removed the financial incentive to keep patients in the hospital longer, leading to significant reductions in hospital patients' lengths of stay (Guterman and Dobson, 1986; Zuckerman et al., 1988). However, studies found that hospitals responded to the new payment system by shifting patients to exempt hospitals (Newhouse and Byrne, 1988) and subsequently to post-acute care facilities that were not included in the DRG payment, causing a spike in the use of home health care and skilled nursing facilities. Quality of care was found not to be impacted by any of these changes (Rogers et al., 1990).

The DRG example demonstrates that providers do respond to payment changes. Many policy makers have further concluded that bundled payment should therefore be broadened to include services from multiple providers (e.g., outpatient and post-acute care providers) because the broader the scope of the bundles, the less latitude there is for substitution (Burton, 2012; Guterman et al., 2009).

Several bundled payment pilots now under way may provide additional evaluation evidence (CMS, 2013b; Hussey et al., 2011). For example, the Center for Medicare and Medicaid Innovation's Bundled Payments for Care Improvement program varies several elements across four models. The first model includes only inpatient care in an acute care hospital for all DRGs, excluding physician services. Hospitals receive a discounted payment but can share any savings with physicians. The second model includes acute inpatient and post-acute care ending either 30 or 90 days after an acute care discharge for selected DRGs. The third model includes only post-acute care beginning within 30 days of an inpatient discharge for selected DRGs. Finally, the fourth model incorporates all care services, including those of a physician, provided during an acute inpatient stay and readmissions. All of these arrangements include shared savings, and participants have considerable discretion in designing payment allocations (CMS, 2013b).

Private-sector payers and providers also are experimenting with bundled payment, and related findings should be relevant to Medicare's pursuit of a long-term payment bundling strategy (Bandell, 2011; Business Wire, 2012; Healthcare Finance News, 2011; Orthopedic & Sports Institute, 2012; SSM Health Care, 2011). For example, Geisinger Health System developed a successful bundled payment program for coronary artery bypass graft surgery (Casale et al., 2007) and has begun implementing bundled payment for additional services (Paulus et al., 2008).

Evaluation literature on bundled payment programs remains scant. In the early 1990s, CMS selected seven hospitals to participate in a bundled payment demonstration for bypass surgery that included all hospital, physician, and other practitioner services provided during a hospital stay plus related readmissions occurring from 3 days to 6 weeks postdischarge. Bundled payments were not adjusted for illness severity. An evaluation of the program showed promising results, with savings of 5 to 10 percent for five hospitals and 20 percent for two hospitals. According to Nelson (2012, p. 20), "Those savings reflect the estimated difference between the bundled payments and the amounts that Medicare would have spent for services provided to those bypass patients in the absence of the demonstration." A systematic review of bundled payment programs found weak but consistent evidence that they reduce costs without adversely impacting quality, although most previous programs have had a more limited scope than the Bundled Payments for Care Improvement program and other recent bundled payment initiatives (Hussey et al., 2012).

Accountable Care Organizations

The ACO is a health care delivery and financing model currently being tested by CMS and commercial insurers. ACO reforms target organized provider organizations and networks that assume responsibility for the quality, cost, and overall care of their patient populations (Correia, 2011; Fisher et al., 2007). ACOs are designed to improve value by giving provider-led organizations a stake in maximizing efficiency within and across delivery settings to meet cost and quality targets. To achieve goals, ACOs might focus on a variety of activities, such as quality improvement, care coordination and discharge processes, protocols for home health referrals, favoring efficient providers for referrals, or targeting high-risk individuals for disease management programs. ACOs are expected to emphasize initiatives most effective in lowering the cost of care and improving outcomes for their populations (Guterman et al., 2011; Nelson, 2012; Share and Mason, 2012).

ACOs vary in structure, ranging from fully integrated health care organizations to networks of hospital(s) and independent primary care and specialty physicians (CMS, 2013d). However, ACOs must meet a base level of organizational capacity in order to assume their responsibilities. Recognizing that ACOs need to have adequate organizational capacity, CMS and private payers call for these health care delivery systems to have (1) a sufficient number of primary care clinicians providing care for a minimum number of beneficiaries, (2) data systems for monitoring and evaluating quality and cost, (3) processes promoting evidence-based medicine, and (4) the ability to receive and distribute performance-based payments (Muhlestein, 2013).

ACOs resemble managed care organizations, but typically are provider organizations rather than traditional insurers.[9] Under Medicare, ACO beneficiaries are not restricted to using ACO-affiliated physicians or facilities; rather, they have full access to all providers accepting Medicare (CMS, 2013a). In the private-sector ACOs, however, the design of insurance benefits steers patients to affiliated providers. For example, health maintenance organization (HMO) plans restrict patients to plan providers, while preferred provider organization (PPO) plans allow for out-of-network service but with higher cost sharing for patients who receive care from out-of-network providers. Medicare ACO providers will need similar incentives to encourage patients to receive their care within network (Van Citters et al., 2012).

CMS currently has three programs promoting ACOs: the Pioneer ACO Model program, the Medicare Shared Savings Program (MSSP), and the Advanced Payment Models ACOs. There are currently 269 health care delivery organizations participating in these programs—32 in the Pioneer ACO Model program, 222 in the MSSP, and 15 in Advanced Payment Model ACOs—reaching more than 4 million Medicare beneficiaries (CMS, 2013h). The three programs differ primarily in the degree of financial risk health care delivery systems agree to assume; plans can choose a payment option that gives them larger rewards when they reduce expenditures if they also agree to accept losses when Medicare expenditures are too high.

Additionally, several states are exploring the possibility of forming ACOs for their Medicaid populations. Medicaid ACO programs vary by state, and are thought to be influenced by the state's managed care experience. Examples include Massachusetts's capitated, multipayer model and Vermont's community-based ACO model (Kaiser Commission on Medicaid and the Uninsured, 2012). Oregon has launched an initiative involving ACO-like coordinated care organizations and currently has 15 such organizations operating in the state (Oregon.gov, 2013).

As indicated earlier, the ACO concept has been adopted by the private sector as well; in fact, more than 150 private-sector ACOs were in existence or in the planning stages prior to the launch of CMS's Pioneer ACO Model program (Muhlestein, 2013). Many provider organizations have entered into contractual relationships with private payers to implement payment approaches resembling the MSSP. Other health care organizations have

---

[9]Much like insurers, however, an ACO may and often will contract with physician groups on either a risk or fee-for-service basis, as indeed the FHS example discussed earlier illustrates.

entered into contracts with private payers, such as Blue Cross Blue Shield of Massachusetts's Alternative Quality Contract, under global payment[10] (Song and Landon, 2012) or other arrangements (e.g., partial capitation[11] and bundled payment) (Muhlestein, 2013). Finally, in recent years, multiple stakeholders (e.g., payers, providers, employers, local governments) have formed region- or community-based "collaboratives" focused on improving the value of health care for their populations. Like ACOs and other integrated organizations, such collaboratives vary in size and structure and may or may not align with traditional geographic units. Thus, they are distinct from geographic areas targeted by a geographically based value index. Box 4-1 presents selected examples of these collaboratives.

Given that the ACO concept is new, evidence demonstrating its impact is sparse. Studies on CMS's Physician Group Practice Demonstration (PGPD), the model for the ACA's ACO provisions, found substantial heterogeneity in results across demonstration sites and population subgroups. One study found that on average, the PGPD saved a mean of $114 annually per beneficiary assigned to a multispecialty physician group in 1 of 10 ACO demonstration sites. However, "Among dually eligible beneficiaries, PGPD physician groups achieved a mean annual per capita savings of $532, or 5%, while savings among non-dually eligible beneficiaries were not statistically significant" (Colla, 2012, p. 1020). Unfortunately, neither the overall results nor even the dually eligible results are likely to be statistically significant when one accounts for heterogeneity among organizations.[12] Another study determined that all 10 participating multispecialty groups met at least 29 of 32 quality measures, yet only 5 of the groups generated Medicare savings, totaling $38.7 million. Further, just one group (Marshfield Clinic) earned more than half of the $31.7 million that was returned to the physician groups (Iglehart, 2010).

One study examined Blue Cross Blue Shield of Massachusetts's ACO-style Alternative Quality Contract (Song and Landon, 2012). The authors found that although the program improved quality scores and produced savings of 2.8 percent over its first 2 years, additional payments (e.g., shared savings and infrastructure) to groups exceeded the savings. Because this program was designed for implementation over a 5-year period and because the savings in the final years are expected to be larger, it may be premature to judge the program's ultimate success.

---

[10]Under global payment, an ACO is at financial risk for all of the items and services covered.

[11]Under partial capitation payment, an ACO is at financial risk for some, but not all, of the items and services covered (Center for Healthcare Quality and Payment Reform, 2010).

[12]The authors did not cluster standard errors on organization, but the results among the dually eligible population in the 10 organizations in the demonstration spanned a wide range, from an estimated savings of $2,499 per dual-eligible at the low end to a cost of $598 at the high end. In 4 of the 10 organizations studied, costs increased for the dually eligible.

BOX 4-1
Multistakeholder Community-Based Collaboratives

Much like accountable care organizations (ACOs) or other integrated organizations, multistakeholder community-based collaboratives may implement a vast range of initiatives, such as those designed to improve data collection and dissemination, promote efficient health care delivery, and provide financial incentives for high-value care (Alliance for Health Reform, 2013; Sennett et al., 2011). Examples of these collaboratives include those found in the Agency for Healthcare Research and Quality's (AHRQ's) learning network for chartered value exchanges and the Brookings Institution's evaluation of three community-based reforms in care for chronic conditions:

- *AHRQ's learning network for chartered value exchanges* since 2007 has brought together 24 community multistakeholder collaboratives from 22 states across the country representing 124 million lives. Thirteen of these collaboratives are statewide programs, while the rest have a substate or regional focus. The value exchanges' main mission is to improve quality and transparency through public reporting of quality and efficiency measurement, provider and consumer incentives, and collaborative leadership (AHRQ, 2011).
- *The Primary Care Information Project* in New York City is an electronic health record adoption and data exchange initiative designed to improve access to preventive services in the ambulatory care setting, primarily for prevention of chronic diseases among the city's underserved (PCIP, 2013).
- *Vermont's Blueprint for Health* is a statewide medical home program for patients with chronic conditions (Vermont.gov, 2013).
- *The Wisconsin Health Information Organization* is a statewide initiative designed to create an all-payer database with which to track health care costs and quality measures, data that can be used to improve the value of care for Wisconsinites with chronic diseases (Wisconsin Health Information Organization, 2013).

Given differences in population demographics, health information technology and other health service infrastructure, and resources among communities, regions, and states, collaboratives differ in their stated health objectives, their chosen initiatives, and the robustness of their interventions (Sennett et al., 2011). To the extent that these community or regional efforts can demonstrate that they improve value, however, payment incentives could be directed toward these collaboratives.

Dual-Eligible Care Integration Demonstrations

The more than 9 million Americans who are eligible for both Medicare and Medicaid benefits account for a disproportionate share of Medicare expenditures: Although they constitute 18 percent of traditional Medicare beneficiaries, they account for 31 percent of Medicare spending (MedPAC, 2012b). Differences between Medicare and Medicaid policies associated with provider reimbursement, beneficiary benefits, and financial incentives result in a health care delivery system more fragmented and uncoordinated for this population than for other Medicare beneficiaries. In April 2011, CMS provided grants to 15 states to undertake care integration initiatives for dual-eligible populations (states will test capitated and/or managed fee-for-service models). One goal of the demonstrations is to determine which care integration and payment models are most effective in improving the quality and efficiency of care for this heterogeneous population. According to the Medicare Payment Advisory Commission (MedPAC, 2012b, p. 63), "The demonstrations are also an opportunity to test how to tailor capitated and [fee-for-service] overlay models to different subgroups of dual-eligible beneficiaries."

The Future of New Payment Reform Models

By creating the Center for Medicare and Medicaid Innovation, the ACA generated a thousand pilot demonstrations of new payment models. It is too early to know which of these models will prove to control health care costs and improve quality. As illustrated by the examples provided above, evidence supporting the effectiveness of new payment models such as VBP, PCMH, bundled payment, and ACOs in controlling costs and improving health outcomes is limited (GAO, 2011; Petersen et al., 2006; Rosenthal, 2008; Scott et al., 2011; Werner et al., 2011). Results of such efforts have been uneven; in the PGPD, for example, 5 of 10 provider organizations achieved CMS's required cost savings to collect bonuses (Iglehart, 2010). Because these models are still in the early stages of development, however, it is critical that CMS continue to evaluate them and use the results to refine their design (IOM, 2012; The National Commission on Physician Payment Reform, 2013). In the interim, the new payment models require payers and providers to make decisions about major design elements despite the lack of adequate evidence to guide those decisions. They must decide (1) which quality and cost indicators to use, (2) how large incentives should be in absolute terms and relative to provider revenue, (3) which services to include in bundles (for bundled payment), and (4) how to assign beneficiaries to particular providers or provider organizations (Miller, 2007). As McClellan (2011, p. 75) noted, "As capacity to measure healthcare processes and outcomes continues to expand rapidly, in conjunction with at least some growing confidence that we are measuring the right things, the linkages between provider payments and measured quality are likely to strengthen."

New payment reforms are designed to reward efficient providers of care and stimulate inefficient providers to improve the care they deliver. In accordance with its statement of task, the committee commissioned RAND Corporation to perform an impact analysis of its recommendations. RAND modeled the impact of pay-for-performance (equivalent to VBP), bundled payment, and ACOs on hospitals, hospital referral regions (HRRs), and total Medicare spending.[13] RAND's analysis demonstrates that payment reforms targeting health care decision makers can result in large changes (by design) in payments to providers within HRRs, even if those reforms do not substantially affect geographic variation in spending among HRRs. In the case of VBP, for example, payment redistributions had no impact on geographic variation, largely because there was no relationship between performance on the quality measures and Medicare spending. The bundled payment policy, however, did reduce geographic variation in Medicare spending since high-spending providers (for selected bundles) were in areas with high overall Medicare spending. Some providers/health systems will flourish with these new incentives; others will struggle, particularly in the first few years (Haywood and Kosel, 2011). It is also likely that local market factors (e.g., population demographics, provider competition) will influence providers' abilities to handle the new payments (Guterman et al., 2011; Pollack and Armstrong, 2011; Werner, 2010); thus, models suited for some areas will face greater challenges in others.

Finally, although some disruption to the current system is inevitable and even warranted, it is critical that Medicare beneficiaries' access to medical care not be diminished. As reforms transition from pilot demonstrations to broader programs, CMS will need to monitor Medicare beneficiaries' access to care.

RECOMMENDATION 4: During the transition to new payment models, the Centers for Medicare & Medicaid Services (CMS) should conduct ongoing evaluations of the impact on value of the reforms included in Recommendation 3 by measuring Medicare spending and beneficiaries' clinical health outcomes. CMS should use the results of these evaluations to iteratively improve these payment models. CMS

---

[13]Time constraints limited the scope of RAND's work to these three payment reforms. Further, given that the committee's research did not yield recommendations on the specifics of payment reforms, the committee did not comment further on the many scenarios modeled by RAND. RAND's report can be accessed at www.iom.edu/geovariationmaterials.

should also monitor how these reforms impact Medicare beneficiaries' access to medical care.

ENCOURAGING BROADER ADOPTION OF NEW PAYMENT REFORMS

If evaluations of pilot reforms demonstrate improvements in value, the next step will be generalization of the reforms to broader populations. Congress might direct the Secretary of Health and Human Services to make the reforms mandatory for all (or a subset of) health care providers that accept Medicare patients. Alternatively, Congress might direct CMS to encourage providers to accept the new payment models through lower updates for traditional Medicare than for new payment models. Translating pilot programs into national policy will be a challenge (Chernew and Goldman, 2013; Greenwald, 2011). As stated earlier, new payment models require major investments in infrastructure (e.g., HIT systems, care managers) if it is to be managed effectively (Korda and Eldridge, 2011). If the new models were mandated before a majority of health care providers had developed the required infrastructure, many organizational failures (e.g., bankruptcies) might result, negatively affecting Medicare beneficiaries' access to care. Similarly, provider organizations will accept new payment models voluntarily only if they believe that bonuses or shared savings will be sufficient to cover their investment in the infrastructure required to achieve efficiencies (Pham et al., 2010). Particularly in the beginning, therefore, Congress might avoid prescribing an immediate wholesale change in payment, instead directing CMS to accelerate the adoption of payment reforms by authorizing differential payment updates for new payment models and traditional Medicare (Davis and Guterman, 2007). It should also be noted that providers serving disproportionately low-income populations may face especially difficult challenges in accessing the necessary resources and may require additional funding to build the organizational capacity to transition to the new payment models (Pollack and Armstrong, 2011; Werner, 2010).

Additionally, Congress should give CMS the flexibility to experiment with the mix of payment mechanisms, rates, and performance metrics that will align provider incentives with high-value care. For example, CMS might test a blended model for payment to PCMHs that combines fee-for-service payments, per-member-per-month (PMPM) care coordination fees, and bonuses for meeting quality and efficiency metrics (e.g., generic prescribing, reduced emergency department use, better management of selected chronic conditions) (Davis and Guterman, 2007). While evaluations are ongoing, CMS should be allowed to alter the levels and payment rates within models to determine those that are most effective.

RECOMMENDATION 5: If evaluations of specific payment reforms demonstrate increased value, Congress should give the Centers for Medicare & Medicaid Services the flexibility to accelerate the transition from traditional Medicare to new payment models.

REFERENCES

Advocate Health Care. 2013. *2013 value report: Clinical integration program evolution.* http://www.advocatehealth.com/clinical-integration-program-overview (accessed July 18, 2013).

AHRQ (Agency for Healthcare Research and Quality). 2011. *Overview: AHRQ learning network for chartered value exchanges.* http://www.ahrq.gov/professionals/quality-patient-safety/quality-resources/value/lncveover.html (accessed July 10, 2013).

Alliance for Health Reform. 2013. *Select community quality initiatives map.* http://allhealth.org/community-initiatives.asp (accessed February 19, 2013).

American Hospital Association. 2010a. *Accountable care organization synthesis report.* Washington, DC: American Hospital Association.

————. 2010b. *Clinical integration—The key to real reform.* Washington, DC: American Hospital Association.

American Medical Association. 2012. *Bundled payments.* http://www.ama-assn.org/ama/pub/physician-resources/practice-management-center/claims-revenue-cycle/managed-care-contracting/evaluating-payment-options/bundled-payments.page (accessed July 18, 2013).

Audet, A.-M. J., M. M. Doty, J. Shamasdin, and S. C. Schoenbaum. 2005. Measure, learn, and improve: Physicians' involvement in quality improvement. *Health Affairs* 24(3):843-853.

Bandell, B. 2011. *Blue Cross signs first bundled payment deal with Miami firm.* http://www.bizjournals.com/southflorida/print-edition/2011/04/08/blue-cross-signs-first-bundled.html?page=all (accessed June 18, 2013).

Bodenheimer, T. 2008. Coordinating care—A perilous journey through the health care system. *New England Journal of Medicine* 358(10):1064-1071.

Burns, L. R., and R. W. Muller. 2008. Hospital-physician collaboration: Landscape of economic integration and impact on clinical integration. *Milbank Quarterly* 86(3):375-434.

Burton, R. 2012. *Improving care transitions.* http://www.rwjf.org/content/dam/farm/reports/issue_briefs/2012/rwjf401314 (accessed July 18, 2013).

Business Wire. 2012. *21st Century Oncology and Humana break new ground with case rate reimbursement agreement.* http://www.businesswire.com/news/home/20120808006089/en/21st-Century-Oncology-Humana-Break-Ground-Case (accessed June 18, 2013).

Campbell, S. M., D. Reeves, E. Kontopantelis, B. Sibbald, and M. Roland. 2009. Effects of pay for performance on the quality of primary care in England. *New England Journal of Medicine* 361(4):368-378.

Casale, A. S., R. A. Paulus, M. J. Selna, M. C. Doll, A. E. Bothe, Jr., K. E. McKinley, S. A. Berry, D. E. Davis, R. J. Gilfillan, B. H. Hamory, and G. D. Steele, Jr. 2007. "Proven-CareSM": A provider-driven pay-for-performance program for acute episodic cardiac surgical care. *Annals of Surgery* 246(4):613-621; discussion 621-613.

Casalino, L., R. R. Gillies, S. M. Shortell, J. A. Schmittdiel, T. Bodenheimer, J. C. Robinson, T. Rundall, N. Oswald, H. Schauffler, and M. C. Wang. 2003. External incentives, information technology, and organized processes to improve health care quality for patients with chronic diseases. *Journal of the American Medical Association* 289(4):434-441.

Cassidy, A. 2010. *Patient-centered medical homes.* http://www.healthaffairs.org/healthpolicy/briefs/brief.php?brief_id=25 (accessed July 18, 2013).

Cebul, R. D., J. B. Rebitzer, L. J. Taylor, and M. E. Votruba. 2008. Organizational fragmentation and care quality in the U.S. healthcare system. *Journal of Economic Perspectives* 22(4):93-113.

Cebul, R. D., T. E. Love, A. K. Jain, and C. J. Hebert. 2011. Electronic health records and quality of diabetes care. *New England Journal of Medicine* 365(9):825-833.

Center for Healthcare Quality and Payment Reform. 2010. *Using partial capitation as an alternative to shared savings to support accountable care organizations in Medicare.* http://www.chqpr.org/downloads/PartialCapitationPaymentforACO.pdf (accessed July 18, 2013).

Chernew, M., and D. Goldman. 2013. Transitioning to bundled payments in Medicare. In *15 ways to rethink the federal budget.* Washington, DC: The Hamilton Project. Pp. 12-16.

Chuang, K. H., H. S. Luft, and R. A. Dudley. 2004. The clinical and economic performance of prepaid group practice. In *Toward a 21st century health system: The contributions and promise of prepaid group practice*, edited by A. C. Enthoven and L. A. Tollen. San Francisco, CA: Jossey-Bass. Pp. 45-60.

CMS (Centers for Medicare & Medicaid Services). 2012. *Pioneer accountable care organization model: General fact sheet.* http://innovation.cms.gov/Files/fact-sheet/Pioneer-ACO-General-Fact-Sheet.pdf (accessed July 18, 2013).

———. 2013a. *Accountable care organizations (ACO).* http://www.cms.gov/Medicare/Medicare-Fee-for-Service-Payment/ACO/index.html?redirect=/aco (accessed July 18, 2013).

———. 2013b. *Bundled payments for care improvement (BPCI) initiative: General information.* http://innovation.cms.gov/initiatives/bundled-payments (accessed July 18, 2013).

———. 2013c. *Comprehensive primary care initiative.* http://innovation.cms.gov/initiatives/comprehensive-primary-care-initiative (accessed May 23, 2013).

———. 2013d. *Fast facts—All Medicare shared savings program and Medicare pioneer ACOs.* http://www.cms.gov/Medicare/Medicare-Fee-for-Service-Payment/sharedsavingsprogram/Downloads/PioneersMSSPCombinedFastFacts.pdf (accessed July 10, 2013).

———. 2013e. *FQHC advanced primary care practice demonstration.* http://innovation.cms.gov/initiatives/FQHCs (accessed May 23, 2013).

———. 2013f. *More doctors, hospitals partner to coordinate care for people with Medicare: Providers form 106 new accountable care organizations.* http://www.cms.gov/apps/media/press/release.asp?Counter=4501&intNumPerPage=10&checkDate=&checkKey=&srchType=1&numDays=3500&srchOpt=0&srchData=&keywordType=All&chkNewsType=1%2C2%2C3%2C4%2C5&intPage=&showAll=&pYear=&year=&desc=&cboOrder=date (accessed July 18, 2013).

———. 2013g. *Multi-payer advanced primary care practice.* http://innovation.cms.gov/initiatives/Multi-Payer-Advanced-Primary-Care-Practice (accessed May 23, 2013).

———. 2013h. *Shared savings program: Program news and announcements.* http://www.cms.gov/Medicare/Medicare-Fee-for-Service-Payment/sharedsavingsprogram/News.html (accessed July 18, 2013).

Colla, C. H. 2012. Spending differences associated with the Medicare physician group practice demonstration. *Journal of the American Medical Association* 308(10):1015-1023.

Correia, E. W. 2011. Accountable care organizations: The proposed regulations and the prospects for success. *American Journal of Managed Care* 17(8):560-568.

Davis, K., and S. Guterman. 2007. Rewarding excellence and efficiency in Medicare payments. *Milbank Quarterly* 85(3):449-468.

Decker, S. L., E. W. Jamoom, and J. E. Sisk. 2012. Physicians in nonprimary care and small practices and those age 55 and older lag in adopting electronic health record systems. *Health Affairs* 31(5):1108.

Dolan, E., and D. Yanagihara. 2011. *Value based pay for performance in California.* Issue brief no. 4. Oakland, CA: Integrated Healthcare Association.

Doran, T., E. Kontopantelis, J. M. Valderas, S. Campbell, M. Roland, C. Salisbury, and D. Reeves. 2011. Effect of financial incentives on incentivised and non-incentivised clinical activities: Longitudinal analysis of data from the UK Quality and Outcomes Framework. *British Medical Journal* 342:d3590.

Enthoven, A. 2009. Integrated delivery systems: The cure for fragmentation. *American Journal of Managed Care* 15:S284-S290.

Fendrick, A. M., and M. E. Chernew. 2006. Value-based insurance design: Aligning incentives to bridge the divide between quality improvement and cost containment. *American Journal of Managed Care* 12 Spec no. SP5-SP10.

Fisher, E. S., D. O. Staiger, J. P. W. Bynum, and D. J. Gottlieb. 2007. Creating accountable care organizations: The extended hospital medical staff. *Health Affairs* 26(1):w44-w57.

Folsom, A., C. Demchak, and S. B. Arnold. 2008. *Rewarding results pay-for-performance: Lessons for Medicare.* http://www.hcfo.org/pdf/monograph0308.pdf (accessed July 18, 2013).

Frakt, A. B., and R. Mayes. 2012. Beyond capitation: How new payment experiments seek to find the "sweet spot" in amount of risk providers and payers bear. *Health Affairs* 31(9):1951-1958.

GAO (Government Accountablility Office). 2011. *Value in health care: Key information for policymakers to access efforts to improve quality while reducing costs.* Washington, DC: GAO.

Gaynor, M., J. B. Rebitzer, and L. J.Taylor. 2001. *Incentives in HMOs.* Cambridge, MA: National Bureau of Economic Research.

Goldberg, D. G., S. S. Mick, A. J. Kuzel, L. B. Feng, and L. E. Love. 2013. Why do some primary care practices engage in practice improvement efforts whereas others do not? *Health Services Research* 48(2, pt. 1):398-416.

Greenwald, L. M. 2011. Converting successful Medicare demonstrations into national programs. In *Pay for performance in health care: Methods and approaches*, edited by J. Cromwell, M. G. Trisolini, G. C. Pope, J. B. Mitchell and L. M. Greenwald. Research Triangle Park, NC: Research Triangle Institute. Pp. 315-340.

Guterman, S., and A. Dobson. 1986. Impact of the Medicare prospective payment system for hospitals. *Health Care Financing Review* 7(3):97-114.

Guterman, S., and H. Drake. 2010. *Developing innovative payment approaches: Finding the path to high performance.* New York: The Commonwealth Fund.

Guterman, S., K. Davis, S. Schoenbaum, and A. Shih. 2009. Using Medicare payment policy to transform the health system: A framework for improving performance. *Health Affairs* 28(2):w238-w250.

Guterman, S., S. C. Schoenbaum, K. Davis, C. Schoen, A.-M. J. Audet, K. Stremikis, and M. A. Zezza. 2011. *High performance accountable care: Building on success and learning from experience.* New York: The Commonwealth Fund.

Hastings, D. 2012. *Medicare ACOs: The integration of financial and clinical integration.* http://healthaffairs.org/blog/2012/04/11/medicare-acos-the-integration-of-financial-and-clinical-integration (accessed July 18, 2013).

Haywood, T. T., and K. C. Kosel. 2011. The ACO model—A three-year financial loss? *New England Journal of Medicine* 364(14):e27.21-e27.23.

Healthcare Finance News. 2011. *Caromont Health and BCBSNC announce bundled payment program for knee replacement.* http://www.healthcarefinancenews.com/press-release/caromont-health-and-bcbsnc-announce-bundled-payment-program-knee-replacement (accessed June 18, 2013).

Herrin, J., B. da Graca, D. Nicewander, C. Fullerton, P. Aponte, G. Stanek, T. Cowling, A. Collinsworth, N. S. Fleming, and D. J. Ballard. 2012. The effectiveness of implementing an electronic health record on diabetes care and outcomes. *Health Services Research* 47(4):1522-1540.

Holroyd-Leduc, J. M., D. Lorenzetti, S. E. Straus, L. Sykes, and H. Quan. 2011. The impact of the electronic medical record on structure, process, and outcomes within primary care: A systematic review of the evidence. *Journal of the American Medical Informatics Association* 18(6):732-737.

Hussey, P. S., M. S. Ridgely, and M. B. Rosenthal. 2011. The PROMETHEUS bundled payment experiment: Slow start shows problems in implementing new payment models. *Health Affairs* 30(11):2116-2124.

Hussey, P. S., A. W. Mulcahy, C. Schnyer, and E. C. Schneider. 2012. Bundled payment: Effects on health care spending and quality closing the quality gap: Revisiting the state of the science. In *Evidence Report/Technology Assessment Number 208. AHRQ Publication No. 12-E007-EF*.

Iglehart, J. K. 2010. Assessing an ACO prototype—Medicare's physician group practice demonstration. *New England Journal of Medicine* 364(3):198-200.

IOM (Institute of Medicine). 2012. *Best care at lower cost: The path to continuously learning health care in America*. Washington, DC: The National Academies Press.

Jackson, G. L., B. J. Powers, R. Chatterjee, J. P. Bettger, A. R. Kemper, V. Hasselblad, R. J. Dolor, R. J. Irvine, B. L. Heidenfelder, A. S. Kendrick, R. Gray, and J. W. Williams, Jr. 2013. The patient-centered medical home: A systematic review. *Annals of Internal Medicine* 158(3):169-178.

James, J. 2012. *Pay-for-performance. New payment systems reward doctors and hospitals for improving the quality of care, but studies to date show mixed results*. http://health affairs.org/healthpolicybriefs/brief_pdfs/healthpolicybrief_78.pdf (accessed July 18, 2013).

Jamoom, E., P. Beatty, A. Bercovitz, D. Woodwell, K. Palso, and E. Rechtsteiner. 2012. Physician adoption of electronic health record systems: United States, 2011. *NCHS Data Brief* 98:1-8.

Jha, A. K., K. Joynt, J. Orav, and A. Epstein. 2012. The long-term effect of premier pay for performance on patient outcomes. *New England Journal of Medicine* 366:1606-1615.

Kaiser Commission on Medicaid and the Uninsured. 2012. *Emerging Medicaid accountable care organizations: The role of managed care*. Washington, DC: Kaiser Family Foundation.

Kern, L. M., A. Wilcox, J. Shapiro, R. V. Dhopeshwarkar, and R. Kaushal. 2012. Which components of health information technology will drive financial value? *American Journal of Managed Care* 18(8):438-445.

Korda, H., and G. N. Eldridge. 2011. Payment incentives and integrated care delivery: Levers for health system reform and cost containment. *Inquiry* 48(4):277-287.

Landon, B. E., I. B. Wilson, and P. D. Cleary. 1998. A conceptual model of the effects of health care organizations on the quality of medical care. *Journal of the American Medical Association* 279(17):1377-1382.

Lindenauer, P. K., D. Remus, S. Roman, M. B. Rothberg, E. M. Benjamin, A. Ma, and D. W. Bratzler. 2007. Public reporting and pay for performance in hospital quality improvement. *New England Journal of Medicine* 356(5):486-496.

Lochner, K. A., and C. S. Cox. 2013. Prevalence of multiple chronic conditions among Medicare beneficiaries, United States, 2010. *Preventing Chronic Disease* 10:E61.

Maeng, D. D., J. Graham, T. R. Graf, J. N. Liberman, N. B. Dermes, J. Tomcavage, D. E. Davis, F. J. Bloom, and G. D. Steele, Jr. 2012. Reducing long-term cost by transforming primary care: Evidence from Geisinger's medical home model. *American Journal of Managed Care* 18(3):149-155.

Mayes, R., and R. A. Berenson. 2006. *Medicare prospective payment and the shaping of U.S. health care*. Baltimore, MD: The Johns Hopkins University Press.

McClellan, M. 2011. Reforming payments to healthcare providers: The key to slowing healthcare cost growth while improving quality? *Journal of Economic Perspectives* 25(2):69-92.

McWilliams, J. M., M. E. Chernew, A. M. Zaslavsky, P. Hamed, and B. E. Landon. 2013. Delivery system integration and health care spending and quality for Medicare beneficiaries. *JAMA Internal Medicine* 173(15):1439-1444.

Mechanic, R., and D. E. Zinner. 2012. Many large medical groups will need to acquire new skills and tools to be ready for payment reform. *Health Affairs* 31(9):1984-1992.

MedPAC (Medicare Payment Advisory Commission). 2012a. Medicare and the health care delivery system. In *Report to the Congress: June 2012*. Washington, DC: MedPAC.

———. 2012b. Medicare payment policy. In *Report to the Congress: March 2012*. Washington, DC: MedPAC.

Miller, H. D. 2007. *Creating payment systems to accelerate value-driven health care: Issues and options for policy reform*. Washington, DC: The Commonwealth Fund.

———. 2011. *Testimony of Harold D. Miller*. http://democrats.energycommerce.house.gov/sites/default/files/image_uploads/Testimony_Miller_05.05.11_SGR.pdf (accessed July 18, 2013).

Moullec, G., K. L. Lavoie, K. Rabhi, M. Julien, H. Favreau, and M. Labrecque. 2012. Effect of an integrated care programme on re-hospitalization of patients with chronic obstructive pulmonary disease. *Respirology* 17(4):707-714.

Muhlestein, D. 2013. *Continued growth of public and private accountable care organizations*. http://healthaffairs.org/blog/2013/02/19/continued-growth-of-public-and-private-accountable-care-organizations (accessed July 18, 2013).

Mullen, K. J., R. G. Frank, and M. B. Rosenthal. 2008. *Can you get what you pay for? Pay-for-performance and the quality of healthcare providers*. Cambridge, MA: National Bureau of Economic Research.

NCQA (National Committee for Quality Assurance). 2011. *New NCQA standards take patient-centered medical homes to the next level*. http://www.ncqa.org/Newsroom/2011NewsArchives/NewsReleaseJanuary282011.aspx (accessed July 10, 2013).

Nelson, L. 2012. *Lessons from Medicare's demonstration projects on disease management and care coordination*. Washington, DC: Congressional Budget Office.

Newhouse, J. P., and D. J. Byrne. 1988. Did Medicare's prospective payment system cause length of stay to fall? *Journal of Health Economics* 7(4):413-416.

Oregon.gov. 2013. *Coordinated care organizations*. http://www.oregon.gov/oha/ohpb/pages/health-reform/ccos.aspx (accessed July 18, 2013).

Orthopedic & Sports Institute. 2012. *Anthem Blue Cross and Blue Shield and Orthopedic & Sports Institute of the Fox Valley announce bundled payment*. http://www.osifv.com/component/content/article/269-bundled-payment.html (accessed June 18, 2013).

Painter, M. W. 2013. *Bundled payments: This way toward a challenging yet better place*. Newtown, CT: Health Care Incentives Improvement Institute.

Partnership for Sustainable Health Care. 2013. *Strengthening affordability and quality in America's health care system*. Washington, DC: Robert Wood Johnson Foundation.

Paulus, R. A., K. Davis, and G. D. Steele. 2008. Continuous innovation in health care: Implications of the Geisinger experience. *Health Affairs* 27(5):1235-1245.

PCIP (Primary Care Information Project). 2013. *Primary Care Information Project.* http:// www.nyc.gov/html/doh/html/hcp/pcip.shtml (accessed July 10, 2013).

Petersen, L. A, L. D. Woodward, T. Urech, C. Daw, and S. Sookanan. 2006. Does pay-for-performance improve the quality of health care? *Annals of Internal Medicine* 145(4): 265-272.

Pham, H. H., D. Schrag, A. S. O'Malley, B. Wu, and P. B. Bach. 2007. Care patterns in Medicare and their implications for pay for performance. *New England Journal of Medicine* 356(11):1130-1139.

Pham, H. H., A. S. O'Malley, P.B. Bach, C. Saiontz-Martinez, D. Schrag. 2009. Primary care physicians' links to other physicians through Medicare patients: The scope of care coordination. *Annals of Internal Medicine* 150(4):236-242.

Pham, H. H., P. B. Ginsburg, T. K. Lake, and M. Maxfield. 2010. *Episode-based payments: Charting a course for health care payment reform.* Washington, DC: National Institute for Health Care Reform.

Pollack, C. E., and K. Armstrong. 2011. Accountable care organizations and health care disparities. *Journal of the American Medical Association* 305(16):1706-1707.

Reid, R. J., K. Coleman, E. A. Johnson, P. A. Fishman, C. Hsu, M. P. Soman, C. E. Trescott, M. Erikson and E. B. Larson. 2010. The group health medical home at year two: Cost savings, higher patient satisfaction, and less burnout for providers. *Health Affairs* 29(5): 835-843.

Rogers, W. H., D. Draper, K. L. Kahn, E. B. Keeler, L. V. Rubenstein, J. Kosecoff, and R. H. Brook. 1990. Quality of care before and after implementation of the DRG-based prospective payment system. A summary of effects. *Journal of the American Medical Association* 264(15):1989-1994.

Rosenthal, M. B. 2008. Beyond pay for performance—Emerging models of provider-payment reform. *New England Journal of Medicine* 359(12):1197-1200.

Rosenthal, M., R. G. Frank, Z. Li, and A. M. Epstein. 2005. Early experience with pay-for-performance: From concept to practice. *Journal of the American Medical Association* 294(14):1788-1793.

RWJF (Robert Wood Johnson Foundation). 2012. *Health policy snapshot: Health care quality.* Princeton, NJ: RWJF.

Ryan, A. M., J. Blustein, and L. P. Casalino. 2012. Medicare's flagship test of pay-for-performance did not spur more rapid quality improvement among low-performing hospitals. *Health Affairs* 31(4):797-805.

Scott, A., P. Sivey, D. Ait Ouakrim, L. Willenberg, L. Naccarella, J. Furler, and D. Young. 2011. The effect of financial incentives on the quality of health care provided by primary care physicians. *Cochrane Database of Systematic Reviews* 9:CD008451.

Sennett, C., K. Matsuoka, S. L. Kocot, M. B. McClellan, and M. Chidester. 2011. *Evaluating community-based reforms in care for chronic conditions: A multi-payer template for information technology initiatives.* Washington, DC: Brookings Institution.

Share, D. A., and M. H. Mason. 2012. Michigan's physician group incentive program offers a regional model for incremental "fee for value" payment reform. *Health Affairs* 31(9):1993-2001.

Share, D. A., D. A. Campbell, N. Birkmeyer, R. L. Prager, H. S. Gurm, M. Moscucci, M. Udow-Phillips, and J. D. Birkmeyer. 2011. How a regional collaborative of hospitals and physicians in Michigan cut costs and improved the quality of care. *Health Affairs* 30(4):636-645.

Shih, A., K. Davis, S. C. Schoenbaum, A. Gauthier, R. Nuzum, and D. McCarthy. 2008. *Organizing the U.S. health care delivery system for high performance.* New York: The Commonwealth Fund.

Shortell, S. M., R. R. Gillies, and D. A. Anderson. 1994. The new world of managed care: Creating organized delivery systems. *Health Affairs (Millwood)* 13(5):46-64.

Song, Z., and B. E. Landon. 2012. Controlling health care spending—The Massachusetts experiment. *New England Journal of Medicine* 366(17):1560-1561.

SSM Health Care. 2011. *Anthem Blue Cross and Blue Shield in Missouri and SSM Health Care-St. Louis collaborate on payment innovation.* http://www.ssmhealth. com/030911anthemorthopayment (accessed June 18, 2013).

Sterns, J. B. 2007. Quality, efficiency, and organizational structure. *Journal of Health Care Finance* 34(1):100-107.

Stremikis, K., C. Schoen, and A. K. Fryer. 2011. A call for change: The 2011 Commonwealth Fund survey of public views of the U.S. health system. *Issue Brief (Commonwealth Fund)* 6:1-23.

The National Commission on Physician Payment Reform. 2013. *Report of the National Commission on Physician Payment Reform.* http://physicianpaymentcommission.org/ wp-content/uploads/2013/03/physician_payment_report.pdf (accessed July 18, 2013).

Van Citters, A. D., B. K. Larson, K. L. Carluzzo, J. N. Gbemudu, S. A. Kreindler, F. M. Wu, S. M. Shortell, E. C. Nelson, and E. S. Fisher. 2012. *Four health care organizations' efforts to improve patient care and reduce costs.* Washington, DC: The Commonwealth Fund.

Vermont.gov. 2013. *Blueprint for health.* http://hcr.vermont.gov/blueprint (accessed July 10, 2013).

Werner, M. 2012. *Physician leadership as an essential capability for transformation and accountable care.* Minneapolis, MN: Fairview Health Services.

Werner, R. M. 2010. Does pay-for-performance steal from the poor and give to the rich? *Annals of Internal Medicine* 153(5):340-341.

Werner, R. M., and R. A. Dudley. 2012. Medicare's new hospital value-based purchasing program is likely to have only a small impact on hospital payments. *Health Affairs* 31(9):1932-1940.

Werner, R. M., J. T. Kolstad, E. A. Stuart, and D. Polsky. 2011. The effect of pay-for-performance in hospitals: Lessons for quality improvement. *Health Affairs* 30(4):690-698.

Wisconsin Health Information Organization. 2013. *The Wisconsin Health Information Organization.* http://www.wisconsinhealthinfo.org (accessed July 10, 2013).

Wolfson, D., E. Bernabeo, B. Leas, S. Sofaer, G. Pawlson, and D. Pillittere. 2009. Quality improvement in small office settings: An examination of successful practices. *BMC Family Practice* 10(1):1-12.

Zuckerman, S., J. Feder, and J. Hadley. 1988. Hospital responses to Medicare's prospective payment system. *Bulletin of the New York Academy of Medicine* 64(1):52-62.

Appendix A

Glossary

Clinical health outcome: A health state of a patient resulting from health care.

Cluster: In this study, various regression models were used to test the influence of a specific "cluster" or group of independent or predictor variables on dependent or outcome variables.

Coefficient of variation (CV): The ratio of the standard deviation of a random variable to its mean. The committee uses the CV to compare the degree of variability in Medicare and commercial populations with respect to health care spending and use. Because both the numerator and the denominator of this variable are in the same units, the magnitude of the CV does not depend on the units in which it is measured (e.g., dollars or thousands of dollars).

Cohort: A group of persons who have at least one clinical characteristic in common. This study defined 15 cohorts based on clinical conditions. A single person may appear in one or more cohorts.

Control model: A statistical model that includes all independent predictor variables, except those an investigator especially wants to understand. In this study, the control regression model is adjusted or controls for length of time beneficiaries are in plans and year of analysis. The effect of other predictors can be calculated by comparing the estimates of models adjusted for clusters 1 through 10 to the control model. In effect, the control model is used to eliminate variation that is of no interest.

Correlation coefficient (Pearson's and Spearman's): A measure of the relationship between two variables, indicating how the direction and magnitude of change in one is accompanied by change in another. It varies between +1 (perfect, positive association, meaning as one variable increases the other variable increases) and −1 (perfect, negative association, meaning as one variable increases the other decreases). It does not, however, indicate that there is a causal relationship between the variables.

Efficiency: Production and allocation of goods and services that generate the most utility for a given set of resources or inputs.

Health care cost: The actual costs of production.

Mean: The average of a group of values.

Median: The value that separates the highest 50 percent of scores on a variable from the lowest 50 percent.

Medicare Part A: Also known as the Hospital Insurance (HI) program, Part A covers inpatient hospital services, skilled nursing facility, home health, and hospice care.

Medicare Part B: Also known as the Supplementary Medical Insurance (SMI) program, Part B helps pay for physician, outpatient, home health, and preventive services.

Medicare Part C (Medicare Advantage): Also known as the Medicare Advantage program, Part C allows beneficiaries to enroll in a private plan, such as a health maintenance organization, preferred provider organization, or private fee-for-service plan, as an alternative to the traditional fee-for-service program. These plans receive payments from Medicare to provide Medicare-covered benefits, including hospital and physician services, and in most cases, prescription drug benefits.

Medicare Part D: Part D, the outpatient prescription drug benefit, was established by the Medicare Modernization Act of 2003 (MMA) and launched in 2006. The benefit is delivered through private plans that contract with Medicare: either stand-alone prescription drug plans (PDPs) or Medicare Advantage prescription drug (MAPD) plans.

Outliers: Values for a variable so extreme that they may have undue influence on the resulting values of certain statistics. They can distort the mean value, but the median value remains unaffected.

Percentile: The value of a variable, below which a certain percentage of data points or observations fall. For example, if Medicare spending at the 90th percentile is $10,000 per person, then 90 percent of all observations would be expected to have spending less than $10,000 per person.

Price: The amount paid by insurers and beneficiaries to a provider for health care services.

Quality: The degree to which health care services for individuals and populations increase the likelihood of patient-desired health outcomes and are consistent with current professional knowledge.

Quintile: One-fifth of a sample or population based on division in intervals of a particular variable. In the Acumen Growth Analysis, hospital referral regions (HRRs) were classified into quintiles based on expenditure levels in 1992, such that the same number of HRRs are included in each quintile. Quintiles are generally presented in order from top to bottom.

Regression analysis: A statistical technique for predicting the value of an dependent variable Y as a function of one or more predictor variables X. The resulting predicted value is the expected value used to calculate the residual.

Residual: The difference between the actual observation (e.g., actual spending in a hospital referral region [HRR]) and the expected value (e.g., expected spending) based on a set of predictor variables. For example, adjusting for mortality in an HRR for its age and sex mix, the residual is the difference between actual mortality and predicted mortality.

Total health care spending: What medical providers and suppliers are paid for their services and products, reflecting both price and utilization of health care services.

Utility: Consumer satisfaction or use.

Utilization: The volume or amount of health care services consumed within a given time period.

Value: The excess (or shortfall) of overall health benefit and/or well-being produced net of health care cost.

Value index: A relative measure of value, e.g., a measure of improvement in patient-centered, clinical health outcomes per unit of resources use in one area relative to the national average.

Appendix B

Acronyms and Abbreviations

AAMC	Association of American Medical Colleges
ACA	Affordable Care Act
ACO	accountable care organization
ACS	American Community Survey
BCBSMA	Blue Cross Blue Shield of Massachusetts
CBO	Congressional Budget Office
CBSA	core based statistical area
CHD	coronary heart disease
CHF	congestive heart failure
CMS	Centers for Medicare & Medicaid Services
COPD	chronic obstructive pulmonary disease
CPT	current procedural terminology
DME	direct medical education or durable medical equipment
DRG	diagnosis-related group
DSH	disproportionate share hospital
FHS	Fairview Health Services
FISMA	Federal Information Security and Management Act of 2002
FQHC	federally qualified health center
GDP	gross domestic product

GPCI	geographic practice cost index
HCC	hierarchical condition category
HEDIS	Health Care Effectiveness Data and Information Set
HHS	U.S. Department of Health and Human Services
HIT	health information technology
HMO	health maintenance organization
HRR	hospital referral region
HRSA	Health Resources and Services Administration
HSA	hospital service area
IHA	integrated health association
IME	indirect medical education
IOM	Institute of Medicine
IQI	inpatient quality composite indicator
MedPAC	Medicare Payment Advisory Commission
MSA	metropolitan statistical area
NCQA	National Committee for Quality Assurance
OIG	U.S. Office of the Inspector General
PCMH	primary care medical home or patient-centered medical home
PCP	primary care physician
PDI	pediatric quality indicator
PGPD	physician group practice demonstration
PHE	precision health economics
PPO	preferred provider organization
PQI	prevention quality indicator
PSI	patient safety indicator
PYE	partial-year enrollment
RVU	relative value unit
RxHCC	prescription drug hierarchical condition category
SGR	sustainable growth rate
VBP	value-based purchasing

Appendix C

Summary of Empirical
Modeling Methodology

The committee commissioned a body of empirical analyses to examine geographic variation in spending, utilization, and quality using public and commercial datasets. The goals of the analyses were to characterize and account for the presence and magnitude of geographic variation across different geographic units, payers, and clinical condition cohorts. The population-specific studies conducted by Acumen, LLC, The Lewin Group, and Harvard University were carried out using the research framework outlined in Table C-1.[1] Precision Health Economics' methodological approach in synthesizing these results and evaluating geographic variation in total health spending is then summarized. The complete methodological details are available in the subcontractor reports.[2]

---

[1]This table only presents the methodology for the Medicare 2007-2009 analysis and does not show the Medicaid 2007-2009 analysis, the Medicare 1992-2010 growth analysis, or the Medicare Advantage 2007-2009 analysis, all of which use variations on this methodological approach.

[2]In addition to the studies summarized in Appendix C, the committee also commissioned reports from the University of Pittsburgh and the Dartmouth Institute for Health Policy and Clinical Practice. All papers can be accessed through the Institute of Medicine website via the following link: http://www.iom.edu/geovariationmaterials.

TABLE C-1
Acumen, Lewin, and Harvard's Study Approach and Methodology in the Medicare and Commercial Analyses

	Acumen	Lewin	Harvard
Data Source	Medicare Analysis: (Parts A, B, and D) Claims and Enrollment data *Medicare Advantage (MA) (Part C) was analyzed separately	Optum De-identified Normative Health Information (dNHI) Database	Thomson Reuters MarketScan Commercial Claims and Encounters database
Years of Analysis	2007-2009	2007-2009	2007-2009
Study Population	• 100% sample of all Medicare fee-for-service beneficiaries • Majority of sample are over age 65. The clinical condition cohort analyses were limited to ages 18 and older. • Excludes costs for beneficiaries in the months that they are enrolled in Medicare Advantage (Part C). Excludes all beneficiaries who have any third-party payment in the observation window.	• Included enrollees between the ages 0-64, with a small sample over age 65. • The clinical condition cohort analyses were limited to ages 18-64.	• Included enrollees between the ages 0-64. • The clinical condition cohort analyses were limited to ages 18-64.
Treatment of "Capitated Claims"	• Not applicable	• Excluded observations (0.3% of population)	• Imputed value (6% of population)
Measurement of Spending	• Total all-cause spending includes all costs incurred by Medicare and the patient in covering inpatient, outpatient, hospice, home health, skilled nursing, carrier, durable medical equipment and Part D claim types. • Medicare analysis follows input-price standardization methodology developed with CMS as	• Total all-cause spending includes all costs of all facility, provider and prescription drug costs incurred by payer, secondary payer and patient. • See Harvard input-price adjustment memo (Appendix E)	• Total all-cause spending includes all costs of all medical and prescription drug costs incurred by payer, secondary payer, and patient. • See Harvard input-price adjustment memo (Appendix E)

133

	part of the Hospital Value Based Purchasing (HVBP) program. • The inpatient claims exclude indirect medical education (IME) and disproportionate share (DSH).		
Measurement of Utilization	Measured in two ways: • Counts per service • Input price-standardized cost (*separate input and output price adjustment is unnecessary in this analysis, as Medicare sets final prices accounting for regional variation*).	Measured in two ways: • Counts per service • Output-price standardized cost (Harvard output-price adjustment memo, Appendix E.3).	Measured in two ways: • Counts per service • Output-price standardized cost (Harvard output-price adjustment memo, Appendix E.3)
Measurement of Quality	• Follows the Agency for Healthcare Research and Quality methodology for analyzing quality • The aggregate quality composites include 8 PSI, 6 IQI, and 12 PQI measures. • Separate quality measures computed for 13 of the clinical condition cohorts.	• Aggregate analyses included AHRQ patient safety indicator (PSI) #90, pediatric quality indicator (PDI) #19, inpatient quality indicator (IQI) #91 and prevention quality indicator (PQI) #90. • Cohort quality analyses were limited those with adequate sample sizes, namely coronary heart disease, diabetes, and low back pain.	• Created original composite measures: 4 domains of PQI, PSI, process measures, and readmissions within 30 days of discharge. • Excluded analysis of PDI as these were rare in the dataset.
Multiple Regression Analyses			
Dependent Variables of Spending and Utilization	• OLS Regression without area fixed effects; estimated area level effects as average of residuals from first model estimation • Did not "shrink" estimates	• OLS Regression with area fixed effects:	• OLS Regression without area fixed effects; estimated area level effects as average of residuals from first model estimation (*Sensitivity analysis showed 0.98 correlation to fixed effects model*) • Empirical Bayes framework of "shrinking" estimates used to correct for small sample size variation

continued

TABLE C-1
Continued

	Acumen	Lewin	Harvard
Market Level Analysis	• Used a 2-stage regression method: Step 1: OLS regression without fixed effects. Step 2: First stage estimates of area effects regressed against a set of market-level measures (outlined in Appendix D). • Method comparable to Harvard; see Appendix F: Harvard Market Level Analysis Methodology Memorandum (11.21.12).	• Used Harvard-developed market level measures (Appendix F.1). • Used a 2-stage regression method: Step 1: OLS regression without fixed effects. Step 2: First stage estimates of area effects regressed against a set of market-level measures (outlined in Appendix D). • Used different set of market predictors.	• Used a 2-stage regression method: Step 1: OLS regression without fixed effects. Step 2: First stage estimates of area effects regressed against a set of market-level measures (outlined in Appendix D). • Method comparable to Acumen; see Appendix F: Harvard Market Level Analysis Methodology Memorandum (11.21.12).
Quality Analyses	• Conducted logistic regression for the IQI and PSI, and OLS regression for the PQI composites.	• Conducted logistic regressions for the PSI and PQIs, predicted the outcomes at an individual level and then averaged at area level to produce a rate. • Risk adjusted based on covariates from cluster regressions rather than covariates used in the AHRQ methodology (PHE, p. 12).	• Used logistic models for "rare" quality outcomes, and linear models for all other outcomes. • The rate is risk adjusted by multiplying the ratio of observed to expected outcomes by a reference rate.
Model Specification Clusters	Refer to Appendix D for the complete list of independent variables used by each subcontractor.		
	Correlation Analyses		
"Within" Analysis	• Examines the distribution of the ratios (10th percentile, 90th percentile, min, max, etc.) of the highest-spending to lowest-spending HSAs by HRR	• OLS regression specifications followed. • Wald Test on HSA fixed effects within HRR. Statistical significance indicated intra-regional variation	• Examines the distribution of the ratios (10th percentile, 90th percentile, min, max, etc.) of the highest-spending to lowest-spending HSAs within by HRR

• Also performs an OLS regression	in spending at HSA level not captured by HRR dummy variables • Intra-regional variation examined using CV for HSA PMPM spending.	• Also Performs an OLS regression of HSA average spending on HRR indicator variables, weighted by beneficiary months in each HSA.
"Between" Analysis		
Reported Pearson correlation of: • Medicare beneficiary utilization across clinical condition cohorts • Medicare beneficiary utilization and quality, across condition cohorts and in aggregate population	Reported Pearson and Spearman correlations of: • HRR spending and rankings across clinical condition cohorts • HRR quality and rankings across clinical condition cohorts • Correlation of spending and quality measures	Examines correlations of: • HRR spending and rankings across clinical condition cohorts • Correlation of spending and quality measures • Correlation of quality across cohorts

Precision Health Economics Study Approach and Methodology Summary:

The Precision Health Economics (PHE) report first synthesized and summarized the results from spending, utilization, and quality regression analyses of the population-specific studies conducted by Acumen, Lewin, and Harvard, allowing for easy comparison of findings across public and private payers. In order to examine variation "within" HRRs, PHE conducted a random effects regression of spending at utilization at the HSA level, with the random effects at the HRR level.

Additionally, PHE created a measure of *total health care spending*, attempting to account for the total United States population by including spending for Medicare, Medicaid, commercially insured, and uninsured populations. This measure was created using the following steps:

1. Obtained spending estimates for Medicare, Medicare Advantage (or Medicare managed care), Medicaid, and commercially insured populations from the empirical analyses conducted by Acumen, Lewin, and Harvard.
2. Estimated spending for the uninsured and Medicaid managed care by HRR.
3. Created payer-specific weights to estimate unadjusted, *total health care spending*. The OptumInsight and MarketScan spending data were alternately used as "proxies" for commercial spending.
4. Created two measures of total PMPM spending by HRR, first unadjusted and then adjusted for input prices. Both estimates were adjusted for age, sex, and health status.

PHE conducted OLS regression analysis of *total health care spending* following methods used by other subcontractors in the individual studies.

- Note, for reasons of parsimony, PHE created an index of "health status" rather than using the complete set of HCCs used in the Acumen studies of Medicare and Medicaid.
- The market level analysis was also conducted using a reduced set of market covariates, selected according to several criteria: policy relevance, lack of redundancy, effect size in the population-specific studies, and, finally, the availability of consistent measurement of the predictors across payers.
- Regressions were also weighted by the population in HRRs. The health status predictors were additionally weighted by that population's share of the total HRR population.

Appendix D

Regression Model Specifications with "Clusters" of Predictors

Cluster 1: Partial-year enrollment (PYE), year, pharmacy benefit, age, sex, age–sex interaction (all subcontractors)

Cluster 2: Health status (All subcontractors) – BASELINE MODEL
    a)   PYE, year, pharmacy benefit, age, sex, age–sex interaction
    b)   Health status

Cluster 3: Race (All subcontractors)
    a)   PYE, year, pharmacy benefit, age, sex, age–sex interaction
    b)   Race

Cluster 4: Income (All subcontractors)
    a)   PYE, year, pharmacy benefit, age, sex, age–sex interaction
    b)   Income

Cluster 5: All common beneficiary independent variables (all subcontractors)
    a)   PYE, year, pharmacy benefit, age, sex, age–sex interaction
    b)   Health status
    c)   Race
    d)   Income

Cluster 6: Employer/insurance (Lewin and Harvard only)
- a) PYE, year, pharmacy benefit, age, sex, age–sex interaction
- b) Benefit generosity and payer/plan type (Harvard and Lewin only)
- c) Data source (Harvard only)
- d) Plan size (Lewin only)

Cluster 7: Market (all subcontractors)
- a) PYE, year, pharmacy benefit, age, sex, age–sex interaction
- b) Access to care, payer mix, hospital competition, supply of medical services, % population uninsured, malpractice environmental risk (all)
- c) Physician competition (Harvard and Acumen)
- d) Health professional mix (Lewin and Acumen)
- e) Percentage of Medicare beneficiaries with supplemental insurance
- f) MA/Medicaid penetration (Acumen only)

Cluster 8: Kitchen sink variables (Subcontractors included all independent variables)

All subcontractors
- a) PYE, year, pharmacy benefit, age, sex, age–sex interaction
- b) Race
- c) Income
- d) Health status and comorbidity adjuster
- e) Access to care
- f) Payer mix
- g) Hospital competition
- h) Supply of medical services
- i) % population uninsured
- j) Malpractice environment risk

Harvard additionally adjusted for:
- Health behavior
- Data source
- Payer/plan type
- Benefit generosity
- Physician composition

Acumen additionally adjusted for:
- Medicare and Medicaid dual eligibility status
- Supplemental Medicare insurance
- Fee-for-service or Medicare Advantage
- Part D enrollment

- Percentage of Medicare beneficiaries with supplemental insurance
- MA/Medicaid penetration
- Physician composition
- Health professional mix

Lewin additionally adjusted for:
- Payer/plan type
- Benefit generosity
- Plan size
- Health professional mix

Cluster 9: All common independent variables only (all subcontractors)
a) PYE, year, pharmacy benefit, age, sex, age–sex interaction
b) Race
c) Income
d) Health status and comorbidity adjuster
e) Access to care
f) Payer mix
g) Hospital competition
h) Supply of medical services
i) % population uninsured
j) Malpractice environment risk

Cluster 10: Cluster 1 and Medicare only IVs (*Acumen only*)
a) PYE, year, pharmacy benefit, age, sex, age–sex interaction
b) Medicare and Medicaid dual eligibility status
c) Supplemental Medicare insurance
d) Part D enrollment
e) Fee for service or Medicare Advantage

Appendix E

Harvard University Price Adjustment Memorandums

HARVARD INPUT-PRICE ADJUSTMENT
MEMORANDUM (11.04.11)

Background

The input price adjustment is meant to reflect variation in input prices required to provide care. Harvard uses input price indices developed by the Centers for Medicare & Medicaid Services (CMS) to adjust raw spending.

The input price adjustment is performed separately for each of two claim types: (1) inpatient facility diagnosis-related groups (DRGs) and (2) inpatient professional current professional terminologies (CPTs) and outpatient CPTs. The specifications for each are described below, but for each the unit of analysis is the "claim-day." A "claim-day" is an aggregation of all spending for a given person for a given procedure code for a given claim type (DRG, inpatient CPT, outpatient CPT). For example, a person may have multiple claims for a given code on a given day. We add up the spending for all of the claims for that person for the same code and claim type on the same date (in the case of inpatient stay, we use the admission date) to calculate average spending for the code. For around 15 percent of medical (nondrug) spending, there is an outpatient claim line that is missing a CPT code. For these claims we distribute the spending over claims that do have a CPT on the same day and for the same person according to the proportion of total daily spending each CPT represents. We believe that the outpatient claims that are missing a CPT code are facility payments that have been carved out of the professional payments, and that this procedure reapportions spending. For the purpose of input price adjustment, we treat claims that are missing a CPT code and that do not have any CPT codes on the same day as if they were an inpatient facility claim.

Inpatient Facility (DRGs)

Each claim day with a DRG code is adjusted by the Area Wage Index Values that include the occupational mix adjustment.[1] The wage index data is merged into MarketScan data by county. 69.7% of the claim amount is adjusted by the wage index value, a proportion based on the labor-related share outlined in the Hospital Inpatient Prospective Payment System Final rule.[2] This is the same procedure we perform on any outpatient claims that cannot be apportioned as described above.

$$(0.697 \times \textit{raw claim day amount} / \textit{wage index}) + 0.303 \times \textit{raw claim day amount}$$

Inpatient Professional and Outpatient Claims (CPTs)

Each claim day with a CPT code is adjusted by the fully-implemented relative value unit (RVU)[3] share multiplied by the relevant GPCI.[4] Inpatient professional and outpatient claims incorporate the practice expense **facility** component of the RVU.

$$\textit{Raw claim day amount} / (\%\textit{Work} \times \textit{Work GPCI} + \\ \%\textit{PE (facility)} * \textit{PE GPCI} + \%\textit{MP} \times \textit{MP GPCI})$$

All other claim types (claims without a valid CPT that cannot be allocated to other claims on the same day, durable medical equipment, prescription drugs) are left unadjusted.

---

[1] The wage index file for 2007 can be found at http://www.cms.gov/AcuteInpatientPPS/WIFN/itemdetail.asp?filterType=none&filterByDID=0&sortByDID=3&sortOrder=ascending&itemID=CMS1187403&intNumPerPage=10.

[2] The final rule for fiscal year 2007 can be found at http://www.cms.gov/AcuteInpatientPPS/IPPS/itemdetail.asp?filterType=none&filterByDID=-99&sortByDID=4&sortOrder=ascending&itemID=CMS1229138&intNumPerPage=10.

[3] The RVU lists are based on the October release for each year. 2007 can be found at http://www.cms.gov/PhysicianFeeSched/PFSRVF/itemdetail.asp?filterType=none&filterByDID=-99&sortByDID=1&sortOrder=descending&itemID=CMS1203203&intNumPerPage=1.

[4] The GPCI lists are based on the October release for each year. 2007 can be found at http://www.cms.gov/PhysicianFeeSched/PFSRVF/itemdetail.asp?filterType=none&filterByDID=-99&sortByDID=1&sortOrder=descending&itemID=CMS1203203&intNumPerPage=10.

Capitated Claims

We outline our overall approach to capitated claims in a separate memo. We will input-price adjust the imputed values for capitated claims.

Aggregation

After the spending is adjusted as described above, the adjusted spending (including spending on claims that are left unadjusted) is summed across a person-year. This results in one input-price adjusted value per person per year.

HARVARD CLAIM-DAY METHOD MEMORANDUM (11.04.11)

Background

There are frequent occurrences of multiple claims for a single procedure coded on a single day for a single person. This is due to the way claims are coded by providers and processed by insurers. We believe the vast majority of these claims are not separate events, but a single event coded on multiple claim lines. In addition, about 14 percent of total medical spending (non-drug) has no associated CPT code. The vast majority (>95 percent) of this spending is represented in the outpatient facility file. After exploring these claims with experts at Thomson Reuters, we believe that the majority are facility fees carved out of outpatient claims.

Harvard's Approach

The general approach is to collapse all claims for a specific service (e.g., CPT code), performed on the same day for the same enrollee to 1 claim-day observation. This is the unit of quantity that will be used throughout much of the analysis, such as creating price lists for output price adjustment. Harvard recognizes that this approach will mean sometimes counting 2 distinct procedures performed on the same day as 1 claim day. As a result those days will be codes as having a higher price as opposed to greater quantity.

More detailed methods are described here:

- For inpatient facility claims, all claims coded as the same DRG on the same date of admission for the same person will be collapsed to 1 claim-day. There are no inpatient facility claims that are missing an associated DRG code.
- CPTs are used for inpatient professional, outpatient professional, and outpatient facility claims. There are three components paid

for a CPT claim a work component, a practice expense and a malpractice component. If the service is provided in a facility (which is always the case for inpatient services and may be the case for outpatient services) the practice expense component is reduced and the facility gets paid separately (by DRG in the case of inpatient or CPT in the case of outpatient). We will collapse inpatient professional claims with the same enrollee, day, and procedure code into 1 claim-day observation.

- For outpatient claims we cannot identify if and how the professional and technical components are broken out, and therefore we will collapse outpatient claims with the same procedure code, enrollee, and day into 1 "claim-day" observation, thus rolling together the professional and facility components.

- Around 45,000 outpatient claims (14 percent of total medical spending in 2007) do not have an associated procedure code. For these claims, we apportion spending across all CPT claims that occurred on the same day for each enrollee based on the proportion of spending that each CPT represents on that day. For instance, if $100 lacked a procedure code, and on the same day we observe two CPTs: CPT "A" for $200 and CPT "B" $400, we apportion the $100 based on a 1/3 and 2/3 ratio, respectively. The new value for CPT "A" is $225, and CPT "B" is $475. We run this apportioning step before performing input or output price adjustments, and before imputing capitated claims.

HARVARD OUTPUT-PRICE ADJUSTMENT MEMORANDUM (10.05.12)

Background

The purpose of the output price adjustment is to eliminate the effect of different prices between locations. Harvard's approach is to create a nationalized standard price for each procedure code and type of claim (inpatient DRG, inpatient CPT, and outpatient CPT) based on the national mean payment for each procedure per day it was rendered. This standard price is then applied back to each claim day of the same type. For example, we compute the mean spending per person per day for a specific code for computed tomography (CT) scan (conditional on being greater than zero for that person on that day). We then apply that price to each person day for the same CT code regardless of where they live or what was actually paid.

Trimming Before Calculating the National Mean Price

We do not trim claims other than those with spending less than or equal to zero. We experimented with trimming and found it made the decomposition into price and quantity effects difficult without substantially altering conclusions about aggregate variation.

Types of Claims Included

The output price adjustment is performed for all inpatient and outpatient claims with a procedure code. Claims that do not include a procedure code and that cannot be apportioned to other claims on the same day are left unadjusted. Capitated claim days are omitted when calculating means/ medians. Drug claims are also left unadjusted

Summing Procedure

After the spending is adjusted as described above, the adjusted spending amounts and residual unadjusted spending (drug claims and claims that are missing procedure code after the apportioning step) are summed across a person-year. This results in one output price adjusted value per person per year.

Zero-Dollar and Capitated Claims

We outline our overall approach to capitated claim-days in a separate memo. We will apply an output price adjustment value to all capitated claim days (even those with observed spending of $0). We will not apply an output price adjustment to non-capitated claim days that have $0 spending. This is because we believe capitated claim days with zero dollar spending generally represent procedures that occurred, while non-capitated claim days with zero dollar spending are likely corrections and do not represent actual services.

Appendix F

Harvard Market Variables Memorandum

HARVARD PRICE INDEX MEMORANDUM (12.21.11)

Background

Hospital referral region (HRR)-level price indices will be used for three purposes:

1. To adjust imputed values for capitated claims based on market-level differences in price; and
2. To examine price variation across markets; and
3. To use as an alternative method creating output price adjustment.

Creating the National Standard Price

The national standard price for each procedure code and type of claim (diagnosis-related group or current procedural terminology) is calculated as the national mean payment for each procedure. In order to calculate the national mean payment per procedure, claim-day records were calculated by summing payments across all records with the same Enrollee ID, service date and procedure code. Capitated claims and non-capitated claims with zero-dollar spending are excluded when calculating the national standard price.

This standard (national mean) price is then applied back to each claim-day with the same procedure code. For example, we compute the mean spending per person per day for a specific code for computed tomography

(CT) scan. We then apply that price to each person day for the same CT code (conditional on being greater than zero for that person on that day) regardless of where they live or what amount was actually paid.

Creating a Market Basket

Harvard has proposed using the following services in the market basket:

- Top 100 DRGs, in terms of total non-capitated expenditures in 2007
- Top 100 outpatient CPTs (see below), in terms of total non-capitated expenditures in 2007
- Top 200 DRGs or CPTs (in terms of total non-capitated expenditure) that are not included in the other two categories in 2007

CPT codes are used in both outpatient and inpatient professional settings. In Medicare there are three components paid for a CPT claim: a work component, a practice expense and a malpractice component. If the service is provided in a facility (which is always the case for inpatient services and may be the case for outpatient services) the practice expense component is reduced and the facility is paid separately (by DRG in the case of inpatient or CPT in the case of outpatient). We cannot identify if and how the professional and technical components are broken out, and therefore we will collapse outpatient claims with the same procedure code, enrollee, and day into 1 "claim-day" observation. This will be our unit of quantity, and it will be used to construct the market baskets and when determining the price index.

The Price Index

Each procedure in the market basket is assigned a weight equal to its proportion of total market basket spending (weights sum to 1).

Within each area, every weight is multiplied by the mean price for that procedure in the area and all procedures are summed. This produces a single value specific to each HRR.

$$Index^{HRR^x} = \sum_{i=1}^{n} Mean_i^x * Weight_i$$

$$Weight_i = \frac{Expenditure_i}{Expenditure_{basket}}$$

HARVARD MARKET LEVEL VARIABLES
MEMORANDUM (10.20.11)

Background

Market level variables are defined at different levels of aggregation (i.e., HRR and county). Competition is inherently defined at the HRR level.

However, the following market variables are available at the county level:

- *Percent uninsured:* American Community Survey (ACS) (source); available at the county level, only for 2008 and 2009 (could also use Current Population Survey [CPS] at the state level for 2005-2009)
- *Commercial health maintenance organization and preferred provider organization penetration as well as Medicaid, traditional medicine (TM), and Medicare Advantage penetration:* Interstudy (source)
- *Physician workforce composition:* area resource file (ARF) (source)
- *Malpractice risk:* Centers for Medicare & Medicaid Services (source); malpractice geographic cost index
- *Population density:* ARF (source)

Approach

We will aggregate the county variables to HRR level (which is imperfect), using a crosswalk based on percent of population in the HRR from a given county. We will then regress the fixed effects from the individual level regressions on the market level variables in order to assess relationship between market variables and geographic variation. For hospital service area (HSA) analysis we will use a similar strategy, applying HRR competition to the HSA.

Alternative

We could assign market level variables to individuals based on their county and then include those variables in the individual level regressions. This is not possible for competition measures because they are collinear with fixed effects. We would still need a second HRR level model to relate fixed effects to competition or we would need to use random effects.

Rationale

We prefer the approach suggested because it keeps all market variables together in the analysis and is more straightforward to explain. Sensitivity analysis and descriptive analyses of within HRR variation in county-level variables will reveal whether the county-level variables produce different results.

HARVARD MARKET LEVEL ANALYSIS
METHODOLOGY MEMORANDUM (11.21.12)

Background

A previous memorandum (Market Level Variables Memo) detailed the construction of HRR and HSA market-level measures. The resulting files are attached to the Portal and contain estimates at the HRR (or HSA) level for each measure that is analyzed. The following explains Harvard implementation of this file and the market-level analysis.

Empirical Approach

The market-level file was merged by geographic unit to a file containing estimates of spending, quantity, input-price adjusted spending, and quality derived from regressions (i.e., a file similar to the Subcontractor's Spreadsheet). We then used multiple linear regressions to assess the relationship between various dependent variables and market-level characteristics. Specifically, we regressed a range of market-level measures (outlined in Harvard's Final Report) against spending, quantity, input-price adjusted spending, and certain quality measures. We employed weights according to population size.

Appendix G

Selected Results of the Committee's Commissioned Empirical Analyses

MEDICARE SERVICE CATEGORY UTILIZATION (MONTHLY COST RESIDUAL) BY HRR

To determine the extent to which variation in particular health care services contributes to total variation in Medicare expenditure, the Committee disaggregated price-standardized, risk-adjusted Medicare spending into seven types of services. Table G-1 sorts 306 hospital referral regions (HRRs) by their total monthly adjusted differences from the national mean of spending (also known as residual cost). This table serves as a supplement to Figure 2-5a–h (Medicare Service Category Utilization by Hospital Referral Region), in Chapter 2.[1]

---

[1]Information on other services categories are available on the Acumen Medicare spreadsheets, which can be accessed through the Institute of Medicine website (http://www.iom.edu/geovariationmaterials).

TABLE G-1
Medicare Service Category Utilization (Monthly Cost Residual) by Hospital Referral
Region (HRR)

HRR Name	Total Monthly Adjusted Differences from the National Mean of Spending Across HRRs	Acute Care Monthly Adjusted Differences from the National Mean of Spending Across HRRs	Post-Acute Care Monthly Adjusted Differences from the National Mean of Spending Across HRRs
Rochester, NY	-$174	-$43	-$79
Stockton, CA	-$172	-$41	-$64
Sacramento, CA	-$171	-$52	-$69
Buffalo, NY	-$166	-$46	-$57
Bronx, NY	-$166	-$38	-$89
Santa Cruz, CA	-$158	-$39	-$64
Santa Rosa, CA	-$157	-$61	-$67
Medford, OR	-$156	-$48	-$69
San Francisco, CA	-$153	-$34	-$65
Salem, OR	-$150	-$47	-$58
Albuquerque, NM	-$149	-$52	-$31
Modesto, CA	-$141	-$25	-$80
La Crosse, WI	-$138	-$36	-$68
Bakersfield, CA	-$136	-$26	-$86
Yakima, WA	-$135	-$39	-$70
Eugene, OR	-$134	-$34	-$59
Santa Barbara, CA	-$134	-$59	-$71
Alameda County, CA	-$133	-$24	-$57
Syracuse, NY	-$131	-$41	-$73
Portland, ME	-$130	-$40	-$36
Fresno, CA	-$130	-$34	-$83
Burlington, VT	-$127	-$38	-$58
San Jose, CA	-$126	-$36	-$58
Portland, OR	-$126	-$36	-$57
Binghamton, NY	-$121	-$45	-$71
Elmira, NY	-$117	-$13	-$71
Danville, PA	-$115	-$49	-$25

TABLE G-1
Continued

HRR Name	Total Monthly Adjusted Differences from the National Mean of Spending Across HRRs	Acute Care Monthly Adjusted Differences from the National Mean of Spending Across HRRs	Post-Acute Care Monthly Adjusted Differences from the National Mean of Spending Across HRRs
Minot, ND	-$114	-$21	-$42
Albany, GA	-$112	-$54	-$62
Olympia, WA	-$110	-$33	-$43
Iowa City, IA	-$108	-$14	-$52
Honolulu, HI	-$108	-$28	-$48
Chico, CA	-$104	-$17	-$57
El Paso, TX	-$104	-$48	-$7
Redding, CA	-$104	-$38	-$45
Dubuque, IA	-$103	-$30	-$41
San Bernardino, CA	-$102	-$23	-$26
Springfield, MA	-$102	-$40	-$12
Pueblo, CO	-$101	-$38	-$34
Marshfield, WI	-$101	-$10	-$61
San Mateo County, CA	-$100	-$28	-$48
Charleston, WV	-$100	-$23	-$50
Appleton, WI	-$99	-$34	-$49
Albany, NY	-$97	-$21	-$57
Roanoke, VA	-$96	-$24	-$25
Sayre, PA	-$96	-$11	-$58
Madison, WI	-$95	-$22	-$37
Bangor, ME	-$93	-$20	-$55
Neenah, WI	-$93	-$34	-$52
Rochester, MN	-$93	-$4	-$51
Napa, CA	-$92	-$15	-$80
Providence, RI	-$92	-$30	-$16
Rapid City, SD	-$91	-$22	-$44
Charlottesville, VA	-$91	-$20	-$36

continued

TABLE G-1
Continued

HRR Name	Total Monthly Adjusted Differences from the National Mean of Spending Across HRRs	Acute Care Monthly Adjusted Differences from the National Mean of Spending Across HRRs	Post-Acute Care Monthly Adjusted Differences from the National Mean of Spending Across HRRs
Everett, WA	-$90	-$38	-$47
Bend, OR	-$88	-$36	-$42
Winchester, VA	-$87	-$18	-$42
Tacoma, WA	-$86	-$28	-$36
Grand Junction, CO	-$84	-$33	-$24
Muskegon, MI	-$83	-$54	-$20
San Luis Obispo, CA	-$82	-$42	-$51
Seattle, WA	-$80	-$27	-$38
Fargo, ND/Moorhead, MN	-$80	-$10	-$35
Contra Costa County, CA	-$79	-$11	-$50
Greensboro, NC	-$79	-$33	-$35
Morgantown, WV	-$76	-$11	-$42
Cedar Rapids, IA	-$75	-$14	-$40
Spokane, WA	-$73	-$38	-$40
Des Moines, IA	-$73	-$5	-$56
Bismarck, ND	-$72	-$5	-$60
Erie, PA	-$72	-$25	-$26
Anchorage, AK	-$72	$6	-$62
Lancaster, PA	-$71	-$11	-$22
Columbus, GA	-$67	-$36	-$15
Lebanon, NH	-$65	-$37	-$22
St. Cloud, MN	-$63	-$1	-$45
Green Bay, WI	-$63	-$15	-$37
San Diego, CA	-$63	-$33	-$28
Grand Rapids, MI	-$62	-$21	-$24
Minneapolis, MN	-$61	$4	-$43
Salinas, CA	-$61	$16	-$57

TABLE G-1
Continued

HRR Name	Total Monthly Adjusted Differences from the National Mean of Spending Across HRRs	Acute Care Monthly Adjusted Differences from the National Mean of Spending Across HRRs	Post-Acute Care Monthly Adjusted Differences from the National Mean of Spending Across HRRs
Mason City, IA	-$59	$8	-$67
Wausau, WI	-$59	-$1	-$44
Harrisburg, PA	-$58	-$18	-$21
Springfield, MO	-$58	-$25	-$21
Kingsport, TN	-$57	-$9	-$9
Duluth, MN	-$57	-$2	-$35
Augusta, GA	-$56	-$25	-$33
Missoula, MT	-$56	-$18	-$36
Durham, NC	-$56	-$16	-$37
Altoona, PA	-$55	-$31	$5
Spartanburg, SC	-$54	-$25	-$12
St. Paul, MN	-$53	$13	-$47
Hartford, CT	-$52	-$24	-$10
Johnstown, PA	-$51	-$3	-$6
Norfolk, VA	-$51	-$13	-$36
Manhattan, NY	-$51	-$10	-$86
Sioux City, IA	-$50	$0	-$52
Lynchburg, VA	-$50	$0	-$5
Springdale, AR	-$48	-$6	$7
Marquette, MI	-$45	-$10	-$39
Manchester, NH	-$44	-$27	$3
Colorado Springs, CO	-$43	-$22	-$8
Newport News, VA	-$42	-$22	-$37
Worcester, MA	-$42	-$18	$16
Billings, MT	-$41	$0	-$45
Reading, PA	-$40	-$8	-$6
Arlington, VA	-$39	-$12	-$20

continued

TABLE G-1
Continued

HRR Name	Total Monthly Adjusted Differences from the National Mean of Spending Across HRRs	Acute Care Monthly Adjusted Differences from the National Mean of Spending Across HRRs	Post-Acute Care Monthly Adjusted Differences from the National Mean of Spending Across HRRs
York, PA	-$39	-$16	-$17
Tucson, AZ	-$39	-$9	-$20
Tallahassee, FL	-$37	-$26	-$10
Ogden, UT	-$37	-$61	$25
Boise, ID	-$35	-$41	$7
Davenport, IA	-$35	$8	-$30
South Bend, IN	-$33	-$22	-$7
Sioux Falls, SD	-$33	$15	-$43
Kalamazoo, MI	-$32	$2	-$16
Reno, NV	-$32	-$12	-$21
Allentown, PA	-$32	$13	-$14
Phoenix, AZ	-$31	$4	-$21
Traverse City, MI	-$31	$3	-$40
Huntington, WV	-$31	$4	-$31
Urbana, IL	-$30	$11	-$38
Fort Wayne, IN	-$29	-$20	-$6
New Haven, CT	-$29	-$10	-$10
Asheville, NC	-$29	-$31	-$11
Richmond, VA	-$28	$17	-$22
Scranton, PA	-$27	-$15	$14
Macon, GA	-$27	$3	-$40
Salt Lake City, UT	-$27	-$50	$13
Atlanta, GA	-$27	-$20	-$15
Petoskey, MI	-$26	-$1	-$29
Waterloo, IA	-$26	$2	-$53
Winston-Salem, NC	-$26	-$12	-$22
Ventura, CA	-$24	-$7	-$45

TABLE G-1
Continued

HRR Name	Total Monthly Adjusted Differences from the National Mean of Spending Across HRRs	Acute Care Monthly Adjusted Differences from the National Mean of Spending Across HRRs	Post-Acute Care Monthly Adjusted Differences from the National Mean of Spending Across HRRs
Bloomington, IL	-$24	$0	-$35
Great Falls, MT	-$23	$15	-$36
Columbia, MO	-$23	$22	-$34
Greenville, SC	-$23	-$20	-$6
Springfield, IL	-$22	$15	-$37
Canton, OH	-$22	-$10	-$2
White Plains, NY	-$17	$16	-$44
Denver, CO	-$16	-$20	-$10
Boston, MA	-$15	-$9	$31
East Long Island, NY	-$15	$12	-$54
Milwaukee, WI	-$15	$11	-$20
Bridgeport, CT	-$14	$1	-$31
Jonesboro, AR	-$14	$6	-$10
Palm Springs/ Rancho Mira, CA	-$14	-$12	-$43
Paterson, NJ	-$14	-$2	-$30
Lansing, MI	-$13	$3	-$19
Flint, MI	-$13	$26	-$20
Temple, TX	-$13	-$25	$27
Hickory, NC	-$12	-$22	-$8
Raleigh, NC	-$12	$1	-$25
Peoria, IL	-$11	$20	-$15
Greenville, NC	-$11	$10	-$43
Charlotte, NC	-$11	-$15	-$18
Johnson City, TN	-$10	$12	$3
Casper, WY	-$9	$20	-$24
Florence, SC	-$9	$23	-$39
St. Joseph, MI	-$9	-$6	-$10

continued

TABLE G-1
Continued

HRR Name	Total Monthly Adjusted Differences from the National Mean of Spending Across HRRs	Acute Care Monthly Adjusted Differences from the National Mean of Spending Across HRRs	Post-Acute Care Monthly Adjusted Differences from the National Mean of Spending Across HRRs
Fort Smith, AR	-$8	-$27	$72
Greeley, CO	-$8	$0	-$9
Knoxville, TN	-$8	-$18	$1
Fort Collins, CO	-$7	-$1	-$8
Grand Forks, ND	-$5	$21	-$29
Newark, NJ	-$5	$14	-$39
Joplin, MO	-$4	$25	-$2
Wilkes-Barre, PA	-$4	-$28	$51
Rockford, IL	-$3	$27	-$18
Washington, DC	-$2	$45	-$48
Wilmington, DE	-$1	$21	-$12
Dothan, AL	-$1	$5	$18
Chattanooga, TN	$0	-$11	$18
Muncie, IN	$0	-$21	$9
Rome, GA	$1	-$1	$8
Little Rock, AR	$2	$12	-$2
Sun City, AZ	$3	$10	-$26
Akron, OH	$3	$13	$7
Morristown, NJ	$4	$5	-$16
Lafayette, IN	$4	-$8	$0
St. Louis, MO	$6	$26	-$13
Youngstown, OH	$7	$29	-$1
Philadelphia, PA	$8	$22	-$17
Lawton, OK	$8	$3	$37
New Brunswick, NJ	$9	$21	-$22
Topeka, KS	$10	$1	-$3
Montgomery, AL	$10	-$12	$21

TABLE G-1
Continued

HRR Name	Total Monthly Adjusted Differences from the National Mean of Spending Across HRRs	Acute Care Monthly Adjusted Differences from the National Mean of Spending Across HRRs	Post-Acute Care Monthly Adjusted Differences from the National Mean of Spending Across HRRs
Ridgewood, NJ	$10	$13	-$22
Cape Girardeau, MO	$10	$3	-$21
Cleveland, OH	$11	$14	$20
Idaho Falls, ID	$11	-$24	$6
Jackson, TN	$12	-$5	$42
Lexington, KY	$12	$7	$4
Boulder, CO	$12	-$2	$0
Cincinnati, OH	$13	$4	$6
Paducah, KY	$13	$34	-$5
Memphis, TN	$14	$10	$15
Indianapolis, IN	$15	-$8	$13
Aurora, IL	$15	$26	$11
Toledo, OH	$15	$21	$6
Pittsburgh, PA	$15	$26	$20
Nashville, TN	$15	$2	$21
Columbia, SC	$16	-$4	-$10
Owensboro, KY	$16	$24	-$24
Oxford, MS	$16	$12	$20
Omaha, NE	$17	$25	-$17
Ann Arbor, MI	$17	$11	$12
Provo, UT	$17	-$45	$44
Huntsville, AL	$19	$8	-$1
Los Angeles, CA	$20	$3	-$12
Columbus, OH	$20	$18	$3
Camden, NJ	$20	$20	-$17
Dayton, OH	$21	$16	$10
Birmingham, AL	$22	$12	$23

continued

TABLE G-1
Continued

HRR Name	Total Monthly Adjusted Differences from the National Mean of Spending Across HRRs	Acute Care Monthly Adjusted Differences from the National Mean of Spending Across HRRs	Post-Acute Care Monthly Adjusted Differences from the National Mean of Spending Across HRRs
Waco, TX	$22	-$6	$37
Saginaw, MI	$25	$32	-$4
Savannah, GA	$25	-$6	-$23
Gainesville, FL	$25	$9	$14
Hackensack, NJ	$26	$13	-$21
Lincoln, NE	$27	$11	-$21
Louisville, KY	$27	$19	$13
Charleston, SC	$29	-$3	-$4
Covington, KY	$30	$48	-$1
Kansas City, MO	$30	$16	$9
Tuscaloosa, AL	$33	$41	$26
Evansville, IN	$34	$8	$23
Mesa, AZ	$34	$15	-$6
Salisbury, MD	$36	$61	-$28
Ocala, FL	$36	-$6	$12
Takoma Park, MD	$37	$60	-$42
Pensacola, FL	$37	$9	$17
Wichita, KS	$39	$18	-$9
Tupelo, MS	$40	-$6	$29
Melrose Park, IL	$40	$49	$31
Kettering, OH	$42	$5	$30
Wilmington, NC	$42	-$12	-$19
Ormond Beach, FL	$43	-$18	$31
Orange County, CA	$44	-$5	$4
Odessa, TX	$47	-$16	$80
San Antonio, TX	$47	-$20	$63
Dearborn, MI	$50	$42	$26

TABLE G-1
Continued

HRR Name	Total Monthly Adjusted Differences from the National Mean of Spending Across HRRs	Acute Care Monthly Adjusted Differences from the National Mean of Spending Across HRRs	Post-Acute Care Monthly Adjusted Differences from the National Mean of Spending Across HRRs
New Orleans, LA	$52	-$20	$85
Hinsdale, IL	$55	$42	$29
Hudson, FL	$57	-$5	$42
Lakeland, FL	$57	$9	$46
Chicago, IL	$59	$51	$63
Mobile, AL	$61	$31	$34
Terre Haute, IN	$64	$11	-$3
Tampa, FL	$65	$13	$44
Detroit, MI	$66	$38	$25
Gary, IN	$66	$50	$26
San Angelo, TX	$67	$16	$55
Abilene, TX	$68	$23	$45
Evanston, IL	$69	$24	$29
Elyria, OH	$69	$51	$28
Orlando, FL	$73	$13	$28
Sarasota, FL	$74	-$36	$11
Texarkana, AR	$75	$1	$94
Pontiac, MI	$75	$32	$16
Houma, LA	$76	-$5	$54
Blue Island, IL	$79	$78	$37
Corpus Christi, TX	$85	-$36	$115
Royal Oak, MI	$90	$37	$22
Elgin, IL	$90	$72	$33
Las Vegas, NV	$91	$27	$54
Joliet, IL	$92	$85	$15
Fort Myers, FL	$93	$1	$10
Lubbock, TX	$93	$23	$73

continued

TABLE G-1
Continued

HRR Name	Total Monthly Adjusted Differences from the National Mean of Spending Across HRRs	Acute Care Monthly Adjusted Differences from the National Mean of Spending Across HRRs	Post-Acute Care Monthly Adjusted Differences from the National Mean of Spending Across HRRs
Bradenton, FL	$96	-$10	$32
Tulsa, OK	$97	$17	$87
Gulfport, MS	$97	$52	$52
Baltimore, MD	$98	$135	-$53
Jacksonville, FL	$98	$24	$28
Austin, TX	$100	-$1	$57
Amarillo, TX	$100	$7	$69
Munster, IN	$104	$78	$50
Oklahoma City, OK	$108	$22	$82
Hattiesburg, MS	$108	$17	$60
Longview, TX	$109	$3	$101
Panama City, FL	$109	$26	$39
Bryan, TX	$111	$33	$60
Jackson, MS	$115	$5	$110
Wichita Falls, TX	$115	-$8	$114
Fort Worth, TX	$116	-$7	$113
St. Petersburg, FL	$120	$13	$72
Meridian, MS	$120	-$4	$125
Clearwater, FL	$120	-$13	$81
Harlingen, TX	$123	-$34	$157
Beaumont, TX	$123	-$5	$102
Slidell, LA	$129	$30	$81
Lake Charles, LA	$132	$17	$107
Tyler, TX	$133	-$2	$90
Victoria, TX	$152	$38	$79
Dallas, TX	$159	-$3	$140
Metairie, LA	$163	$11	$111

TABLE G-1
Continued

HRR Name	Total Monthly Adjusted Differences from the National Mean of Spending Across HRRs	Acute Care Monthly Adjusted Differences from the National Mean of Spending Across HRRs	Post-Acute Care Monthly Adjusted Differences from the National Mean of Spending Across HRRs
Fort Lauderdale, FL	$172	-$2	$52
Baton Rouge, LA	$172	-$12	$140
Shreveport, LA	$174	$20	$145
Lafayette, LA	$177	$5	$143
Alexandria, LA	$180	$41	$134
Houston, TX	$189	$23	$120
Monroe, LA	$229	$8	$179
McAllen, TX	$266	-$23	$255
Miami, FL	$435	-$10	$350

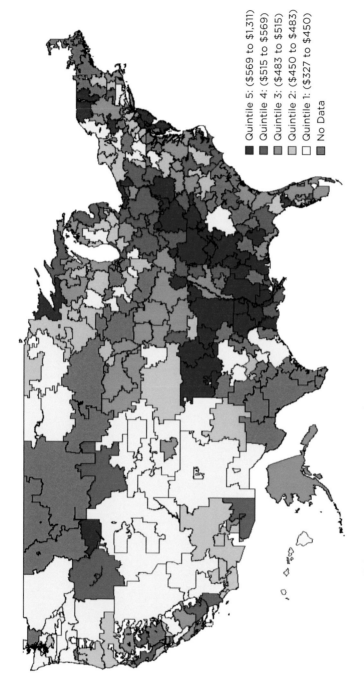

FIGURE G-1 Input-price-adjusted/total health care spending by hospital referral region (HRR).

Quintile 5: ($569 to $1,311)
Quintile 4: ($515 to $569)
Quintile 3: ($483 to $515)
Quintile 2: ($450 to $483)
Quintile 1: ($327 to $450)
No Data

NOTE: PHE's analysis of total health care spending accounts for the commercially insured, Medicare, Medicaid, and the uninsured. HRR regions are divided into five spending quintiles. The figure above illustrates the variation in total health care spending in the United States. Refer to the original subcontractor report for details on methodology, and associated discussion.

SOURCE: PHE, 2013.

Appendix H

Public Workshop Agendas

NOVEMBER 9-10, 2010

20 F Street, NW, Conference Rooms A & B
Washington, DC 20001

DAY 1: TUESDAY, NOVEMBER 9, 2010

10:00 – 10:05   Welcome and Introductory Remarks
Joseph Newhouse, Ph.D., Committee Chair and
Moderator

Policy and Legislative Context for the Study
10:05 – 10:20   Remarks from Study Sponsor, Centers for Medicare &
Medicaid Services (CMS)
Jonathan Blum, Deputy Administrator, Center for
Medicare, CMS, U.S. Department of Health and Human
Services

10:20 – 10:35   Legislative Perspectives
• *The Honorable Allyson Schwartz*, U.S. House of
Representatives

10:35 – 11:30   Legislative Panel Discussion
• *Timothy Gronniger*, Professional Staff, Committee on
Energy and Commerce, U.S. House of Representatives

- *Geoff Gerhardt*, Professional Staff, Subcommittee on Health, Committee on Ways and Means, U.S. House of Representatives
- *Chris Dawe*, Health Counsel, Committee on Finance, U.S. Senate
- *Susan Walden*, Health Policy Counsel, Committee on Finance (Minority), U.S. Senate

11:30 – 12:30   **LUNCH BREAK**

Geographic Variation in Spending and Utilization
12:30 – 1:00   Current MedPAC Research and Experiences
- *Mark Miller, Ph.D.*, Executive Director, MedPAC

1:00 – 1:30   Approaches to Measuring and Interpreting Health Care Variation
- *Michael Chernew, Ph.D.*, Professor, Department of Health Care Policy, Harvard Medical School

1:30 – 2:00   Dartmouth Atlas Research on Variation
- *Jonathan Skinner, Ph.D.*, Joan Sloan Dickey Third Century Professor in Economics, Dartmouth Medical School

Remarks from The Honorable Donald M. Berwick
2:00 – 2:30   Reviewing Geographic Variation as We Improve Health Care Quality
- *Donald M. Berwick, M.D., M.P.P.*, Administrator, CMS, U.S. Department of Health and Human Services

2:30   **Adjourn Open Session**

DAY 2: WEDNESDAY, NOVEMBER 10, 2010

8:00 – 8:05   Welcome and Introductory Remarks
- *Joseph Newhouse, Ph.D.*, Chair and Moderator

Measuring Quality and Value
8:05 – 9:45   Panel Discussion on Measuring Quality and Value
- *Janet Corrigan, Ph.D., M.B.A.*, President and Chief Executive Officer, National Quality Forum

- *Carolyn M. Clancy, M.D.*, Director, Agency for Healthcare Research and Quality, U.S. Department of Health and Human Services
- *Peggy O'Kane, M.S.*, President, National Committee for Quality Assurance
- *Richard Kronick, Ph.D.*, Deputy Assistant Secretary, Office of Health Policy, Office of the Assistant Secretary for Planning and Evaluation, U.S. Department of Health and Human Services

9:45   **Adjourn Open Session**

JANUARY 17, 2011

Keck Center, Room 100
500 Fifth Street, NW
Washington, DC 20001

8:45 – 8:50   Welcome and Introductory Remarks
Joseph Newhouse, Ph.D., Committee Chair and Moderator

Workshop Panels
8:50 – 9:40   Panel 1: *Hospitals/Health Systems*
- Larry Minnix, American Association of Homes and Services for the Aging
- Scott Malaney, American Hospital Association
- Helen Darling, National Business Group on Health, and Bruce Pyenson, Milliman, Inc.

9:40 – 9:45   **BREAK**

9:45 – 10:45 Panel 2: *Clinicians*
- Larry DeGhetaldi, California Medical Association
- John Tooker, American College of Physicians
- Eileen Sullivan-Marx, University of Pennsylvania School of Nursing
- Jonathan Sunshine, American College of Radiology

10:45 – 10:50 **BREAK**

10:50 – 11:50 Panel 3: *Value Commentators*
- Denis Cortese, Arizona State University
- Herbert Pardes, New York Presbyterian Hospital

- Chris Queram, Wisconsin Collaborative for Healthcare Quality

Adjourn Open Session

11:50 – 12:45 **Lunch**
(Committee meets in closed session; guests are encouraged to visit local restaurants for lunch)

OPEN SESSION

12:45 – 1:45 Panel 4: *Consumers and Purchasers*
- Elizabeth Gilbertson, Hotel Employees and Restaurant Employees International Union Welfare Fund
- Lina Walker, AARP
- Sam Nussbaum, WellPoint

PUBLIC TESTIFIERS

1:45 Speakers Begin (*Committee Q&A after each speaker*)
- **John (Jack) Lewin**
  CEO, American College of Cardiology, Washington, DC
- **Deborah Schumann**
  Physicians for a National Health Program, Bethesda, MD
- **Michael Kitchell**
  Iowa Medical Society, Ames, IA
- **Lorrie Kaplan**
  Executive Director, American College of Nurse-Midwives, Silver Spring, MD
- **Jason Scull**
  Program Officer for Clinical Affairs, Infectious Disease Society of America, Arlington, VA
- **James Rohack**
  Director, Scott & White Center for Healthcare Policy, Temple, TX
- **Andrea Weddle**
  Executive Director, HIV Medicine Association, Arlington, VA
- **William Rich**
  Medical Director of Health Policy, American Academy of Ophthalmology, Washington, DC

- **William Davenhall**
  Global Manager, HHS, Esri, Redlands, CA
- **Anne O'Rourke**
  Senior Vice President of Federal Relations, California Hospital Association, Washington, DC
- **Michael Richards**
  Executive Director Government Relations & External Affairs, Gundersen Lutheran Health System, La Crosse, WI
- **Cynthia Flynn**
  General Director, Family Health and Birth Center, Washington, DC
- **Nancy Lane**
  President, PDA Inc. Health Planning Management Consultants, Raleigh, NC
- **Craig Samitt**
  President & CEO, Dean Clinic, Madison, WI
- **Raymond Gibbons**
  Professor of Medicine, Mayo Clinic, Rochester, MN
- **Karl Ulrich**
  President/CEO, Marshfield Clinic, Marshfield, WI
- **Jeffrey Bailet**
  SVP and President of Aurora Medical Group, Milwaukee, WI

Adjourn Open Session

Appendix I

Committee Biographies

Joseph P. Newhouse, Ph.D. (*Chair*), is the John D. MacArthur Professor of Health Policy and Management at Harvard University, Director of the Division of Health Policy Research and Education, chair of the Committee on Higher Degrees in Health Policy, and Director of the Interfaculty Initiative in Health Policy. He is a member of the faculties of the John F. Kennedy School of Government, the Harvard Medical School, the Harvard School of Public Health, and the Faculty of Arts and Sciences, as well as a faculty research associate of the National Bureau of Economic Research. He received B.A. and Ph.D. degrees in economics from Harvard University.

In 1981 Dr. Newhouse became the founding editor of the *Journal of Health Economics*, which he edited for 30 years. He is a current member of the editorial board of the *New England Journal of Medicine*. He has served as the vice-chair of the Medicare Payment Advisory Commission, chaired the Prospective Payment Assessment Commission, and served as a Commissioner of the Physician Payment Review Commission. From 2007 to 2012 he served on the CBO Board of Health Advisers and from 2010 to 2012 he co-chaired the Medicare Trustees Technical Advisory Panel. He has received numerous prizes and awards for his research. He is a director of Aetna, Abt Associates, and the National Committee for Quality Assurance (NCQA).

Alan M. Garber, M.D., Ph.D. (*Vice-Chair*), is Provost of Harvard University and the Mallinckrodt Professor of Health Care Policy at Harvard Medical School, a professor of economics in the Faculty of Arts and Sciences, professor of public policy in the Harvard Kennedy School of Government, and professor in the Department of Health Policy and Management in the

171

Harvard School of Public Health. Before becoming the provost at Harvard, Dr. Garber was the Henry J. Kaiser Jr. Professor and a professor of medicine, as well as a professor of economics, health research and policy, and economics in the Graduate School of Business (by courtesy) at Stanford University. From 1997 to 2011, he was Director of the Center for Primary Care and Outcomes Research in the Stanford University School of Medicine and Director of the Center for Health Policy at Stanford, and from 1986 to 2011 he served as a staff physician at the Department of Veterans Affairs Palo Alto Health Care System. Dr. Garber is an elected member of American College of Physicians, the Association of American Physicians, and the Institute of Medicine of the National Academy of Sciences, and an elected fellow of the Royal College of Physicians. He currently serves as associate editor for the *Journal of Health Economics*. He is a member of the Board on Science, Technology, and Economic Policy of the National Academies and formerly served as a member of the Panel of Health Advisers for the Congressional Budget Office (CBO). Dr. Garber graduated summa cum laude from Harvard College with an A.B. in economics in 1976. He earned an A.M. in economics in 1977 and a Ph.D. in economics in 1982, both from Harvard University. In 1983, he received his M.D. from Stanford University School of Medicine.

Peter Bach, M.D., is the Director of the Center for Health Policy and Outcomes at the Memorial Sloan-Kettering Cancer Center. His main research interests cover health care policy, particularly as relates to Medicare, racial disparities in cancer care quality, and lung cancer epidemiology. His research examining quality of care for Medicare beneficiaries has demonstrated that blacks do not receive as high quality care as whites when diagnosed with lung cancer, and that the aptitude and resources of primary care physicians who treat blacks are inferior, when compared to primary care physicians who primarily treat whites. In 2007 he was the senior author on a study demonstrating that care in Medicare is highly fragmented, with the average beneficiary seeing multiple primary care physicians and specialists. His work in lung cancer epidemiology has focused on the development and utilization of lung cancer prediction models that can be used to determine what lung cancer events populations of elderly smokers will experience over a period of time. His health care policy analysis includes investigations into Medicare's approaches to cancer payment, as well as developing models of alternative reimbursement, payment systems, and coverage policies. He is funded by grants from the National Institute of Aging, a contract from the NCI, and philanthropic sources. He formerly served a senior adviser to the Administrator of the Centers for Medicare & Medicaid Services (CMS). He serves on several national committees, including the Institute of Medicine's National Cancer Policy Forum and the Committee on Performance

Measurement of the NCQA. He chairs the Technical Expert Panel that is developing measures of cancer care quality for CMS. Along with publishing in the medical literature, Dr. Bach's opinion pieces have appeared in numerous lay news outlets, including the *New York Times*, the *Wall Street Journal*, *Forbes Online*, and National Public Radio.

Joseph Baker, J.D., has been president of the Medicare Rights Center since June 2009. Mr. Baker is a member of the Institute of Medicine's Board on Health Care Services and Committee on Geographic Variation in Health Care Spending and Promotion of High-Value Care. He also serves on the CMS Advisory Panel on Outreach and Education. He is an adjunct professor at the New York University School of Law, where he teaches a class on implementation of the Affordable Care Act.

Previously, he was the deputy secretary for health and human services in New York State under Governor David A. Paterson, where he was instrumental in developing Medicaid reforms and a proposal to extend health coverage to younger New Yorkers. Mr. Baker served as assistant deputy secretary for health and human services under Governor Eliot Spitzer, after having directed the Health Care Bureau under Spitzer when he was attorney general of New York. Mr. Baker was executive vice president of Medicare Rights from 1994 to 2001, and prior to that was associate director of legal services for Gay Men's Health Crisis. He is a graduate of the University of Virginia School of Law.

Amber E. Barnato, M.D., M.P.H., M.S., is a tenured associate professor of medicine, clinical and translational science, and health policy and management. She is a board-certified public health and preventive medicine physician and health services researcher whose NIH-funded research focuses on elucidating the determinants of hospital and provider variation in intensive care unit (ICU) and life-sustaining treatment use among elders. She is vice-president elect of the Society for Medical Decision Making and a fellow of the American College of Preventive Medicine, and a former visiting scholar at the CBO. She received her B.A. in physiology from the University of California (UC), Berkeley, her M.D. from Harvard Medical School, her M.P.H. in health policy and management from UC Berkeley, and her M.S. in health services research from Stanford University.

Robert Bell, Ph.D., has been a member of the Statistics Research Department at AT&T Labs-Research since 1998. He previously worked at RAND doing public policy analysis. His current research interests include machine learning methods, analysis of data from complex samples, and record linkage methods. He was a member of the team that won the Netflix Prize competition. He has served on the Fellows Committee of the American

Statistical Association, the board of the National Institute of Statistical Sciences, the Committee on National Statistics, the advisory committee of the Division of Behavioral and Social Sciences and Education, and several previous National Research Council (NRC) advisory committees studying statistical issues, from conduct of the decennial census to airline safety.

Karen Davis, Ph.D., is currently the Eugene and Mildred Lipitz Professor in the Department of Health Policy and Management and director of the Roger C. Lipitz Center for Integrated Health Care at the Bloomberg School of Public Health at Johns Hopkins University. The center strives to discover and disseminate practical, cost-effective approaches to providing comprehensive, coordinated, and compassionate health care to chronically ill people and their families. Dr. Davis has served as president of The Commonwealth Fund, chairman of the Department of Health Policy and Management at The Johns Hopkins Bloomberg School of Public Health, and deputy assistant secretary for health policy in the Department of Health and Human Services (HHS). In addition, she was a senior fellow at the Brookings Institution in Washington, DC, a visiting lecturer at Harvard University and an assistant professor of economics at Rice University. She received her Ph.D. in economics from Rice University

A. Mark Fendrick, M.D., is a professor of internal medicine in the School of Medicine and a professor of health management in the School of Public Health at the University of Michigan. Dr. Fendrick currently directs the Center for Value-Based Insurance Design at the University of Michigan [www.vbidcenter.org], the leading advocate for development, implementation, and evaluation of innovative health benefit plans. Dr. Fendrick's research focuses on the clinical and economic assessment of medical interventions, with special attention to how technological innovation influences clinical practice, benefit design, and health care systems. Dr. Fendrick remains clinically active in the practice of general internal medicine. He is the co–editor in chief of the *American Journal of Managed Care* and is an editorial board member for three additional peer-reviewed publications. He serves on the Medicare Coverage Advisory Committee.

Paul B. Ginsburg, Ph.D., is president of the Center for Studying Health System Change (HSC). Founded in 1995 with support from the Robert Wood Johnson Foundation, HSC conducts research to inform policymakers and other audiences about changes in organization, financing and delivery of care and their effects on people. HSC is widely known for the objectivity and technical quality of its research and its success in communicating it to policy makers, industry and the media as well as to the research community. It enjoys particular respect for its knowledge of developments in communities and health care markets. A sister organization to Mathematica Policy Research, Inc., HSC is funded by the National Institute for Health Care Reform (NIHCR) and various foundations and government agencies. Dr. Ginsburg also serves as research director of NIHCR. See www.hschange. org and www.nihcr.org for additional information.

Prior to his founding HSC, Dr. Ginsburg served as the founding executive director of the Physician Payment Review Commission (now the Medicare Payment Advisory Commission). Widely regarded as highly influential, the Commission developed the Medicare physician payment reform proposal that was enacted by the Congress in 1989. Dr. Ginsburg was a senior economist at RAND and served as deputy assistant director at the CBO. Before that, he served on the faculties of Duke and Michigan State Universities. He earned his doctorate in economics from Harvard University.

Dr. Ginsburg is a noted speaker and consultant on the changes taking place in the health care system and the future outlook. In addition to presentations on the overall direction of change, his recent topics have included cost trends and drivers, consumer-driven health care, provider payment, future of employer-based health insurance, and competition in health care. As a consultant to the Bipartisan Policy Center, he has contributed to reports on reducing federal spending on health care and policies to contain health care costs. He has been named to *Modern Healthcare*'s "100 Most Influential Persons in Health Care" eight times. He received the first annual HSR Impact Award from AcademyHealth. He is a founding member of the National Academy of Social Insurance and a Public Trustee of the American Academy of Ophthalmology, served two elected terms on the Board of AcademyHealth, and serves on the *Health Affairs* editorial board.

Douglas A. Hastings, J.D., currently serves as chair of the Board of Directors of Epstein Becker & Green, P.C., and is based in the Washington, DC, office. He is a member of the firm's Health Care and Life Sciences practice and is a strategic advisor with the firm's consulting affiliate EBG Advisors. Mr. Hastings provides a wide range of health care organizations with strategic and transactional guidance in responding to the challenges and opportunities of the rapidly changing U.S. health care system. He is a graduate of Duke University and the University of Virginia Law School.

Mr. Hastings served on the Board on Health Care Services of the Institute of Medicine (IOM) from 2003 to 2011. He is a member of the National Advisory Board of *Accountable Care News* and a member of the Advisory Board of the *BNA's Health Law Reporter*. He is a past president and fellow of the American Health Lawyers Association and was named one of the nation's "Most Influential Lawyers" by the *National Law Journal* in 2011. In 2010, he was presented with the David J. Greenburg Service Award from the American Health Lawyers Association, was named by *Best Lawyers* as the "Washington, DC Health Care Lawyer of the Year," and received the *BNA Insights* Award for his article, "The Timeline for Accountable Care." He is listed in *Chambers USA Leading Lawyers for Business* in Band 1 for health care transactions nationally.

Brent C. James, M.D., M.Stat., is known internationally for his work in clinical quality improvement, patient safety, and the infrastructure that underlies successful improvement efforts, such as culture change, data systems, payment methods, and management roles. He is a member of the Institute of Medicine (and participated in many of that organization's seminal works on quality and patient safety). He is a fellow of the American College of Physician Executives and holds faculty appointments at the University of Utah School of Medicine, Harvard School of Public Health, and the University of Sydney, Australia, School of Public Health. He is chief quality officer, and executive director, at the Institute for Health Care Delivery Research at Intermountain Healthcare, based in Salt Lake City, Utah. Through the Intermountain Advanced Training Program in Clinical Practice Improvement (ATP), he has trained almost 5,500 senior physician, nursing, and administrative executives, drawn from around the world, in clinical management methods, with proven improvement results.

He has been honored with a series of awards for quality in health care delivery, and for 8 of the 9 years it has been in existence, he has been named among *Modern Physician*'s "50 Most Influential Physician Executives in Healthcare." He has been named among the "100 Most Powerful People in Healthcare" (*Modern Healthcare*) for 5 years, and *Modern Healthcare*'s "25 Top Clinical Informaticists" for the 2 years it has been in existence. Before coming to Intermountain, he was an assistant professor in the Department of Biostatistics at the Harvard School of Public Health, providing statistical support for the Eastern Cooperative Oncology Group (ECOG), and staffed the American College of Surgeons' Commission on Cancer. He holds bachelor of science degrees in computer science (electrical engineering) and medical biology; an M.D. (with residency training in general surgery and oncology); and a master of statistics degree. He serves on several nonprofit boards of trustees dedicated to clinical improvement.

Kimberly S. Johnson, M.D., M.H.S., is an assistant professor of medicine in the Division of Geriatrics and Center for Palliative Care and a fellow in the Center for the Study of Aging and Human Development at Duke University Medical Center. She received her undergraduate education at Dillard University in New Orleans, Louisiana, and her M.D. from Johns Hopkins University School of Medicine. She completed her residency training in internal medicine, fellowship in geriatrics, and clinical research training at

Duke University Medical Center. Dr. Johnson is board-certified in internal medicine, geriatrics, and hospice and palliative medicine.

Dr. Johnson's research focuses on understanding racial disparities in end-of-life care. She has published widely and is nationally recognized for her work investigating how cultural beliefs and preferences and organizational practices and policies may influence the use of hospice care by older African Americans. Dr. Johnson has received the American Academy of Hospice and Palliative Medicine Junior Investigator Award and American Geriatrics Society Outstanding Excellence in Geriatric Research Award for her work. Her research is supported by a Beeson Career Development Award in Aging Research and an R01 from the National Institute on Aging.

Emmett B. Keeler, Ph.D., is a professor at the Pardee RAND Graduate School, an adjunct professor at the University of California, Los Angeles, School of Public Health, and senior mathematician at RAND. In the RAND Health Insurance Experiment, he investigated the theoretical and empirical effects of alternative health insurance plans on episodes of treatment and on health outcomes. The resulting micro-simulation model has been used to study spending and insurance choice. He has led studies to evaluate a new model for helping people with chronic diseases manage their health better and to improve the management of childbirth. He taught at Harvard and the University of Chicago while on leave from RAND. He is the author or co-author of many journal articles, and four books. His research interests are in cost-effectiveness analysis, insurance design, health economics, and health services research. He was the 2003 Distinguished Investigator of AcademyHealth and is a member of the IOM. He received his B.A. from Oberlin College and Ph.D. in mathematics from Harvard University.

Thomas H. Lee, M.D., is an internist and cardiologist and is network president for Partners Healthcare System, the integrated delivery system founded by Brigham and Women's Hospital and Massachusetts General Hospital, and chief executive officer for Partners Community HealthCare. He is a graduate of Harvard College, Cornell University Medical College, and Harvard School of Public Health. He is a professor of medicine at Harvard Medical School and professor of health policy and management at the Harvard School of Public Health. His research interests include risk stratification and optimal management strategies for common cardiovascular problems, and improvement of quality of care, with a particular focus on critical pathways, guideline development and implementation, and managed care.

Dr. Lee is a member of the Board of Directors of Geisinger Health System, the Special Medical Advisory Group of the Department of Veterans Affairs, and the Panel of Health Advisors of the CBO. With James J.

Mongan, M.D., he is the author of *Chaos and Organization in Health Care* (MIT Press, 2009). He is an associate editor of the *New England Journal of Medicine*.

Mark B. McClellan, M.D., Ph.D., is director of the Engelberg Center for Health Care Reform and Leonard D. Schaeffer Chair in Health Policy Studies at the Brookings Institution. Dr. McClellan's work at the Engelberg Center focuses on promoting high-quality, innovative, and affordable health care. A doctor and economist by training, he also has a highly distinguished record in public service and in academic research. Dr. McClellan is a former administrator of the CMS and former commissioner of the U.S. Food and Drug Administration (FDA), where he developed and implemented major reforms in health policy. These include the Medicare prescription drug benefit, FDA's Critical Path Initiative, and public-private initiatives to develop better information on the quality and cost of care. Dr. McClellan chairs the Reagan-Udall Foundation, is co-chair of the Quality Alliance Steering Committee, sits on the National Quality Forum's Board of Directors, is a member of the IOM, and is a research associate at the National Bureau of Economic Research. He previously served as a member of the President's Council of Economic Advisers and senior director for health care policy at the White House and was an associate professor of economics and medicine at Stanford University.

Sally C. Morton, Ph.D., is Professor and Chair of the Department of Biostatistics in the Graduate School of Public Health, and directs the Comparative Effectiveness Research Core at the University of Pittsburgh. She holds secondary appointments in the Clinical and Translational Science Institute, and the Department of Statistics. Previously, she was vice president for statistics and epidemiology at RTI International. She spent the first part of her career at the RAND Corporation, where she was head of the Statistics Group, and held the RAND Endowed Chair in Statistics. Her research interests include the use of statistics in evidence-based medicine, particularly meta-analysis. She serves as an evidence synthesis expert for the Agency for Healthcare Research and Quality Evidence-Based Practice Center (EPC) program, and was co-director of the Southern California EPC. She has been a member of several IOM committees on comparative effectiveness research, and systematic reviews. Dr. Morton is a member of the National Academy of Sciences Committee on National Statistics, Chair of the Statistics Section of the American Association for the Advancement of Science (AAAS), and a statistical expert for the Patient-Centered Outcomes Research Institute (PCORI) Methodology Committee. She was the 2009 president of the American Statistical Association (ASA), is a Fellow of the ASA and of the

AAAS, and is an elected member of the Society for Research Synthesis Methodology. She received a Ph.D. in statistics from Stanford University.

Robert D. Reischauer, Ph.D., is a Distinguished Institute Fellow and president emeritus of the Urban Institute, a nonprofit, nonpartisan policy research and education organization that he was the president of from 2000 to 2012. Between 1989 and 1995, he served as the director of the CBO. He also served as CBO's deputy director, assistant director for Health, Retirement and Long-Term Analysis and executive assistant to the director between 1975 and 1981. Reischauer has been a senior fellow (1986-1989 and 1995-2000) and research associate (1970-1975) in the Economic Studies Program of the Brookings Institution and the senior vice president of the Urban Institute (1981-1986).

Reischauer, who holds an A.B. from Harvard and a master's in international affairs and a Ph.D. in economics from Columbia University, is one of two public trustees of the Social Security and Medicare Trust Funds. He is a founding member of the Academy of Social Insurance and a member of the American Academy of Arts and Science, the IOM, the National Academy of Public Administration, and CBO's Panel of Health Advisers. He was a member of the Medicare Payment Advisory Commission (MedPAC) from 2000 to 2009, serving as its vice chair from 2001 to 2008. He chaired the National Academy of Social Insurance's project, "Restructuring Medicare for the Long Term," from 1995 to 2004. Reischauer, who serves on the boards of several nonprofit organizations, is the senior fellow of the Harvard Corporation.

Alan Weil, J.D., has been the executive director of the National Academy for State Health Policy (NASHP) since September 2004. An independent, nonpartisan, nonprofit research and policy organization, NASHP is dedicated to excellence in state health policy and practice. Prior to joining NASHP, Mr. Weil served as director of the Urban Institute's Assessing the New Federalism project, one of the largest privately funded social policy research projects ever undertaken in the United States. He previously held a cabinet position as executive director of the Colorado Department of Health Care Policy and Financing, was health policy advisor to Colorado Governor Roy Romer, and was assistant general counsel in the Massachusetts Department of Medical Security.

Mr. Weil is a frequent speaker on national and state health policy, Medicaid, federalism, and implementation of the Affordable Care Act. He is the co-editor of two books, publishes regularly in peer-reviewed journals, has testified before Congress more than half a dozen times, and is called on by major media outlets for his knowledge and analysis.

He is on the editorial board of the journal *Health Affairs*, and is a member of IOM's Board on Health Care Services, The Commonwealth Fund's Commission on a High Performance Health System, and the Kaiser Commission on Medicaid and the Uninsured. He is a member of the Board of Trustees of the Consumer Health Foundation in Washington, DC, and of the Board of Directors of the National Public Health and Hospitals Institute. He is a graduate of UC Berkeley, the John F. Kennedy School of Government at Harvard University, and Harvard Law School.

Gail R. Wilensky, Ph.D., is an economist and senior fellow at Project HOPE, an international health foundation. She directed the Medicare and Medicaid programs and served in the White House as a senior adviser on health and welfare issues to President George H. W. Bush. She was also the first chair of the Medicare Payment Advisory Commission. Her expertise is on strategies to reform health care, with particular emphasis on Medicare, comparative effectiveness research, and military health care.

Dr. Wilensky currently serves as a trustee of the Combined Benefits Fund of the United Mine Workers of America and the National Opinion Research Center, is on the Board of Regents of the Uniformed Services University of the Health Sciences (USUHS), the Visiting Committee of the Harvard Medical School, and the Board of Directors of the Geisinger Health System Foundation. She is an elected member of the IOM and has served two terms on its governing council. She is a former chair of the board of directors of Academy Health, a former trustee of the American Heart Association, and a current or former director of numerous other nonprofit organizations. She is also a director of Brainscope, Quest Diagnostics, and United HealthGroup. Dr. Wilensky testifies frequently before congressional committees, serves as an adviser to members of Congress and other elected officials, and speaks nationally and internationally. She received a bachelor's degree in psychology and a Ph.D. in economics at the University of Michigan and has received several honorary degrees.